AGELESS WOMAN

From the Same Author

L'Andropause, cause, conséquences et remèdes

Éditions Maloine, Paris, 1ère édit., 1988

Paris, 2e édit., 1989

Au-delà de cette limite votre ticket est toujours valable

Éditions Albin Michel, Paris, 1991, 1992

El hombre sin edad

HMS WORLD Editions, 2016

L'homme sans âge

HMS WORLD Editions, 2016

Ageless Man

HMS WORLD Editions, 2017

Georges Debled, MD

AGELESS WOMAN

How to Cure and Prevent Diseases of Aging

HMS WORLD

AGELESS WOMAN

How to Cure and Prevent Diseases of Aging

HMS WORLD Editions

www.hmsworld.net

ISBN: 9798648911345

Contents

Part III

Diseases of Aging

Part IV

Revitalize Your Body

Conclusion

Ageless Woman

Author's Note

Sooner or later, starting from age forty, most women will experience various conditions and disorders: general tiredness, overweight, cardiovascular troubles, sexual problems, memory loss, irritability, and a tendency toward depression. Often, they attribute these disturbances to stress and overwork. Such concerns increase after age fifty, the time of menopause.

These disorders are due to a pathological phenomenon that is the start point of sexual aging, reproductive aging, and diseases of aging. I presented on this topic in Madrid in 2015.

For the moment, it is enough for the reader to know that in terms of quantity, the daily production of male hormones in a healthy woman always exceeds the production of female hormones.

Menopause is a nonpathological symptom of a disease. Unfortunately, generally, that disease is not recognized. Some say it does not exist. But that disease has a commencement around age forty—and sometimes before. In women, this condition produces a pathological fall in the production of dihydrotestosterone, the healthy sex hormone, and, consequently, sexual aging. With time, there is also a pathological progressive fall in testosterone that finalizes in deficient testosterone and diseases of aging.

This book explains the mechanisms of an unrecognized disease, *androgenic disease of menopause*, and how to prevent sexual aging and the pathology of aging in women in their early stages. It is impossible to understand the diseases of aging if we do not know how aging appears at its beginning. The prevention of diseases of aging is a priority for everyone. A final note is that some of the references in this book are recent and unpublished. However, they are available to researchers interested in discoveries or new theories.

Medicine of the Twenty-First Century

Medicine is now radically personalized to recognize the singularity of each person. It is possible to analyze the molecule encoding the genetic instructions for each organism. Each treatment can thus be made specific to the individual.

The development of cellular therapy and regenerative medicine will bring about the medical revolution of the twenty-first century: new cells, artificial or reprogrammed, will be produced to regenerate the human body or to replace defective tissues or organs.

With the success of such treatments, it will be necessary to analyze and correct the integrity of testosterone and its metabolism in each human being.

Testosterone is essential for the construction of all organisms' proteins—in both women and men. Consequently, it constitutes one of the bases of metabolism and is the starting point for the prevention of diseases due to aging. Many recent scientific studies confirm this point.

The effects of testosterone on one's metabolism are unique for everyone, man, or woman, and an analysis of these effects is available today. Testosterone production self-destructs during the twenty years preceding death, causing diseases related to aging, so this deterioration must be corrected to avoid these many diseases. I have been addressing this topic for men since 1974, and it has not yet been contradicted and remains relevant. Since 1998, I have demonstrated the same phenomenon in women: the lack of dihydrotestosterone and testosterone production in women produces diseases of aging. I presented on this topic in Madrid in 2015. Beyond age sixty, two out of three women take two types of medicine, and 5 percent of sexagenarians have a form of dementia. States devote colossal sums to "looking after" diseases of aging, which are never cured and thus constitute a bottomless financial drain.

It is necessary to understand the conditions of aging and the mechanisms of degradation so that women will hold their destinies in their own hands.

This book clearly shows one of the fundamental mechanisms that starts the progressive deterioration of the female organism. All organs are involved. By beginning the anti-aging treatment at the onset of the first symptom, often at the age of forty and sometimes even before, it is then possible to avoid diseases of aging. In this book, we will see how the vascular deterioration responsible for Alzheimer's disease can be avoided. The lack of treatment of menopausal androgenic disease causes entire-body degeneration in forty years, thus between ages forty and eighty. In other words, therapy to treat androgenic disease of menopause is a key to prevent diseases of aging.

It will take more than one or two generations for universities to begin teaching about androgenic disease of menopause, but when "medical experts" confirm the existence of a new condition of aging, it is already too late. The preventive treatment must begin forty years before the disasters of old age, mainly because male hormones can currently be accurately measured.

Women over age forty and apparently in good health are actually "sick people" who ignore or are unaware of the degradation of their biochemical body structures, which leads to disease of aging and death around age eighty, in general.

Androgenic disease of menopause is a systemic disease affecting all structures of the body. Today, women over age eighty treated for androgenic disease of menopause on time are looking and feeling age sixty or less and will remain ageless women for dozens of years. Until when? Nobody knows.

The average *healthy* life span in developed countries is sixty-two years, and the average life span is eighty-two years. Securing medical insurance after the age of sixty-five is virtually impossible because insurers cover a random risk and not a certainty. Indeed, the diseases of aging (part III of this book) develop during the last twenty years of life.

Health maintenance is the medicine of the twenty-first century. The art of healing of this era is the art of preventing disease. It is based on the singular analysis of the biology of each person and the particular treatments that this implies: the replacement of missing hormones, the substitution of missing vitamins and minerals, the correction of oxidative stress, and the search for carcinogenic factors and their correction.

Today's medicine deals with diseases by treating them according to traditional medical practice. The vast majority of conditions are due to age. These are the diseases of aging that never get cured despite the constant efforts of health-care workers and specialists.

Shortly, small structures will replace large hospitals, which will close, creating unemployment among the current health professions. Indeed, the prevention of conditions of aging is inexpensive, and with the implementation of prevention, diseases of aging will disappear, as will the bottomless financial traps they create.

The medicine of the twenty-first century already exists. It is evidence-based, preventive, and scientific medicine. It is the heart of a new medical profession.

A reader eager to live a long, healthy life shall find here ways to avoid the shipwreck of old age. Think and act now.

Part I

The Female Climacteric

or

Menopause

1

Sexual and Reproductive Aging Announce Degeneration of All Structures of the Female Body

One day or another, sexual and reproductive regression will reach all women beyond age forty. This phenomenon can also strike young women. The progressive degeneration of the body is the rule after fifty.

Genital aging causes sterility with menopause but also sexual disorders and micturition problems. Sexual motivation disappears, and one's general condition worsens. The end of sexual activity has been accepted less and less by women confronted with a situation for which they do not find any logical explanation.

What they are unaware of, because of a lack of information, is that the male hormone testosterone initially governs the structures of all proteins in the body. All organs consist of proteins, and testosterone controls their assembly. When this vital element has suddenly gone missing because of age, structures degenerate.

Testosterone also acts on the genitals by controlling their development and their integrity; it is the precursor of dihydrotestosterone, the real active sex hormone.

Reduction in the secretion of male hormones consequently provokes not only sexual aging but also a regressive transformation of the body, which one can observe in the following ways:

- An increase in weight, with a progressive heaviness of the silhouette
- Muscular atrophy (testosterone is the muscles' food)

• Brittle bone tissue, followed by rheumatism of the shoulder, osteoarthritis of the spinal column, and so on

• Reduction of memory

• Melancholia and irritability

• General tiredness, anemia

• Development of arteriosclerosis

• Varicose veins in the legs

• Hemorrhoids

• Skin that becomes thin and reddens from the sun rather than browning

• Hypertension, a consequence of arterial hardening

For everyone, the genetic clock starts the process of sexual aging at around forty years old. Individual variations exist, which explains the later aging of certain women, who consequently live longer. There are families in which more former members are still living, and there are different ones in which members die young.

This difference is probably related to the capacity of the sexual glands to secrete more or fewer hormones over time. This phenomenon also explains, among other things, the existence of centenarians.

The gene responsible for sexual aging is not known. On the other hand, the biological characteristics of this regression and their consequences are becoming better known. Consequently, preventive medication exists, and this book aims to explain the preventive approach.

Notwithstanding that women's aging has been the object of constant study for about fifty years, hormone replacement therapy (HRT) has been a disaster.

The traditional definition of menopause signifies the cessation of menstruation. But this is only one symptom among others—the most obvious of which is excess weight and psychological involution. Menopause characterizes the end of one's reproductive life, the start of which begins with puberty and, like it, extends over several years. The word *puberty* was introduced in the fourteenth century. It encompasses all of the physiological and psychological modifications that occur at the time of the passage from childhood to adolescence. In other words, the blossoming of sexuality at the time of puberty accompanies the well-known transformation of this period of life, and sexual regression that appears at the time of menopause accompanies the physical and psychic involution of the body. Although distinct, these phenomena of regression need better understanding.

Women past menopause do not produce ova anymore and are inevitably sterile. Also, they can experience all the disorders of androgenic disease of menopause.

What Are We Talking? A Definition of the Female Climacteric, Menopause, and Androgenic Disease of Menopause

It is helpful first to define the terminology.

Climacteric

The *Collins Dictionary* defines *climacteric* as follows:

noun: 1. a critical event or period; 2. another name for menopause; 3. the period of a man's life corresponding to menopause, chiefly characterized by diminished sexual activity.

Menopause

The word *menopause* goes back to 1823. *Merriam-Webster* gives different meanings for the word, as follows:

a (1): the natural cessation of menstruation usually occurring between the ages of 45 and 55.

(2): the physiological period in the life of a woman in which such cessation and the accompanying regression of ovarian function occurs.

—also called climacteric, climax

—compare perimenopause—the period around the onset of menopause that is often marked by various physical signs (such as hot flashes and menstrual irregularity)

b: cessation of menstruation from other than natural causes (as from surgical removal of the ovaries). Premature menopause due to surgery or ovarian failure.

The first meaning (a-1) of menopause signifies the end of ovarian function, characterized by the stop of ovulation and menstrual bleeding (which are physiological changes).

The second meaning (a-2) refers to the time when menopause occurs—or, more usually, "the female climacteric."

Two meanings for one word make it impossible to identify a disease and, consequently, its treatment.

What is this phenomenon about which we are speaking? It is impossible to understand the diseases of aging if the menopause phenomenon is not understood first. Menopause is a state of aging that presents apparent signs: the stopping of ovulation and the cessation of menstruation; those conditions are physiological and are not a disease.

Menopausal Disease or Androgenic Disease of Menopause

Introduction

To define a new idea is not an easy thing because there is no preliminary reference.

The concept and pathology of "menopausal disease" or androgenic disease of menopause are unknown. The reality of this pathological entity, however, is founded on the following:

• Knowledge of physiology and hormonal biochemistry of the female cycle, found in excellent hormonology treatises (see, e.g., Baulieu and Kelly [1]—a book that every doctor should have read)

• Clinical experience and detailed biochemical analyzes that I began in 1998 in "postmenopausal" women with characteristic symptoms of "menopausal disease" (The initial clinical study was pursued through an appropriate therapeutic attitude when "menopausal disease" was diagnosed biochemically.)

• Results of women treated with mesterolone, which relieved their symptoms (Each chemical analysis here concerns the biochemical and clinical singularity of each woman.)

Menopause

The definition of the word *menopause* is limited to the cessation of menstruation. Therapy for menopause is a meaningless concept because menopause is not a disease.

More than 100,000,000 references on Google use the term *menopause*. *HRT* is also commonly used concerning menopause.

The Terminology of "Menopausal Disease"

The terminology *menopausal disease* corresponds, in linguistics, to a terminological use of collocations. *Menopausal disease* is a collocation. In corpus linguistics, a collocation is a sequence of words or terms that co-occur more often than expected by chance. The term *menopausal disease* has the technical signification that it is a disease. *Menopause* signifies the "cessation of menstruation," and *disease* means the "deterioration of health." I have not found any better terminology than *menopausal disease* because the principal—but nonpathological—symptom is the permanent absence of menstruation; the pathological symptoms are described later in the discussion. I would not mind if an "enlightened mind" should propose a better term for this disease. I also use *androgenic disease of menopause* and *androgenic menopausal disease* throughout this text, which perhaps are more fitting. Those who want to improve the concept are welcome to do so. History will choose.

Androgenic disease of menopause describes the following:

• The **cause:** a reduction of the secretion of androgen hormones (testosterone and dihydrotestosterone) with age

• The **local consequences,** accompanied or not accompanied by **general disorders:** urinary symptoms, sexual symptoms, vasomotor symptoms, psychic symptoms, and constitutional symptoms

• The **specific treatment:** mesterolone, a hormone that acts as dihydrotestosterone (and testosterone), which has only existed since 1967

Androgenic menopausal disease occurs from age forty onward and sometimes before. It appears when the production of androgen hormones (testosterone and dihydrotestosterone) decreases significantly. I propose the following medical definition:

Menopausal Disease* or *Androgenic Disease of Menopause

Menopausal disease is the whole of the pathological and psychopathological modifications brought out by acute or progressive cessation of ovarian production of androgens after the end of menstruation [2].

Explanation of the Definition

I once met a menopausal woman. I was talking about the aging of male genitalia in women, she asked, "What the hell is that?". I replied that the clitoris, the labia majora and labia minora, and the outlet of the bladder are sensitive to dihydrotestosterone, thus constituting the male genital organs of the woman.

In the absence of male hormone, these organs atrophy producing the following symptoms:

- Pain during intercourse
- Insensitive clitoris
- Insensitive vulva
- Urgency to urinate
- Cystitis
- Urinary incontinence
- Reduction in libido

If there are no male genitalia disorders, there is no androgenic disease of menopause. A postmenopausal woman should be aware of this distinction.

The decline in the production of androgens means that the hormone dihydrotestosterone (i.e., the sex hormone) is no longer produced in sufficient quantities through the transformation of testosterone. Testosterone is not the sex hormone; it is transformed into dihydrotestosterone.

If there is no symptom of masculine genitalia disorder, there is no menopausal disease. If there is no menopausal disease, no hormonal treatment is justified.

General Troubles of Androgenic Syndrome or Disease of Menopause

The following disorders may exist in a woman with an androgenic menopausal illness:

- Excess of weight
- Weakness
- Obesity
- Intestinal distension
- Osteoarthritis (shoulder, knee, hip, spinal column)
- Brittleness of the articular ligaments
- Osteoporosis (osseous brittleness, fractures)
- Muscular brittleness
- Hypertension
- Angina pectoris
- Myocardial infarction
- Arteriosclerosis
- Varicose veins
- Hemorrhoids
- Varicose ulcers
- Gangrene
- Anemia
- Thick blood
- Arterial or venous thrombosis
- A rise in blood cholesterol (especially "bad" cholesterol)
- Increase of blood triglycerides
- Diabetes
- Wrinkles
- Thinning hair and dry skin
- Inadequate filtration of the kidneys, leading to uremia

- Immune system deficit, predisposing to cancers
- Vision troubles
- Hearing disorders
- Loose teeth
- Depression, poor self-image, irritability, melancholy, suicidal tendency, incapacity to act
- Chills
- Night sweats
- Sleep problems
- Migraine headaches
- Incapacity to react to stress
- Vaginal dryness

In the months or years leading up to menopause (perimenopause), women might experience the following signs:

- Vaginal atrophy
- Irregular periods
- Sterility from lack of ovulation
- Absence of menstruation
- Uterus atrophy
- Loss of breast fullness

These symptoms are not those of androgenic disease of menopause. These are typically well-known symptoms of gynecological disorders.

Syndromes Mimicking Androgenic Disease of Menopause

When illness exists, different but similar situations may be present. For example, some syndromes* cause the same symptoms as those of menopausal androgenic disease:

- The removal of both ovaries
- When climacteric starts before menopause

Research Findings

A study by Zumoff, Strain, Miller, and Rosner [3] looked at plasma testosterone in the first part of the menstrual cycle in thirty-three women. The average results, reported in the accompanying table, show that the average testosterone levels are 50 percent lower in the forty-year-old woman compared with the twenty-year-old woman, with the decrease in levels worsening with age since the twenties.

Mean Plasma Concentrations of Testosterone before Menopause [3].	
Mean Age	Mean Results (nanogram/mL)
21	0.37
40	0.18

Table 1

Based on Zumoff, Strain, Miller, and Rosner (1995) [3].

---

* A *syndrome* is a series of several symptoms and signs associated with a given condition, which, as allowed by their group, guide diagnosis (Larousse dictionary definition).

My twenty-year clinical experience with plasma levels of testosterone (and dihydrotestosterone) in women proves that these levels continue to decrease after forty years of age, causing disorders such as urgency and urinary incontinence. It is for this handicap that the sales of hygienic protection explode with the aging of populations because both men and women have the same urinary symptoms. In Japan, sales of hygienic protection for adults exceed those for babies. However, it is a medical problem for which there is a treatment.

Researchers from the Department of Obstetrics and Gynecology at the University of Southern California, Los Angeles, have demonstrated the secretion of testosterone by the ovaries after menopause [4]. A gradient for testosterone between the ovarian venous and peripheral blood was present in four of five women who were menopausal for more than ten years [4], explaining why womenfolk have androgenic menopausal disease at different ages.

Androgenic syndrome of menopause is a common disease with a singular treatment. It has nothing to do with the "classic treatment of menopause"—HRT, which is not a treatment but a poisoning by useless proliferative hormones [5].

The diagnosis of androgenic disease of menopause is often simple. Checking testosterone and dihydrotestosterone in the blood is inexpensive. For technical reasons, the treatment uses mesterolone, a safe dihydrotestosterone mimetic. The biochemical results after therapy compared with those before treatment prove the biological improvement linked with the elimination of clinical symptoms (chapter 31).

The time has come to place each doctor at the center of cheap and straightforward therapeutics for androgenic disease of menopause.

2

Male Hormones: Keys to Menopausal Troubles

Hormones are molecules secreted by an organism's glands. When released into the blood, they convey a message or information to a target organ. The cells of the target contain receptors, causing a reaction or signal when they are activated.

The primary role of hormones is to maintain the constancy of the internal environment, which ensures the independence of the organism to the continually changing external world.

By providing communication between cells, hormones integrate biochemical reactions and are essential to the harmonious development of the human body from birth to adulthood.

Other necessary ingredients include vitamins obtained from food, which contrast with hormones, which are only produced by the glands of the organism.

If hormone secretion is defective at birth, the body develops abnormally. When the production of hormones stops in the adult, targets are destroyed, and the body becomes deformed.

Various glands secrete the principal hormones: the pituitary, the thyroid, the adrenals, the pancreas, the ovaries, and the testicles. Each gland secretes specific substances necessary for the regulation and excellent performance of the organism. An excess or deficiency of hormonal secretion causes particular disorders.

The ovaries do not escape the law that governs all the glands. Their secretion of male hormones gradually decreases after the age of twenty. A significant deficiency also occurs after the bilateral removal of the ovaries.

Testosterone: Hormone of a Long, Healthy Life

The ovaries produce ovules and secrete androgen hormones, revealing the masculine sexual characteristics of women. They are released directly into the blood.

Androgens also have general effects necessary to the organism's construction. These effects are particularly spectacular at the time of puberty, which determines the transformation of the small girl into a teenager and then into a complete adult woman.

Testosterone is a principal hormone. Its action is shown in many organs [1]. It is the hormone that governs the construction of proteins present in all structures of the human body.

The skeletal muscle contains receptors for male hormones [2]. In all individuals, there is a relationship between the blood levels of male hormones and the muscular mass. A quite muscular woman has a masculine appearance as a result of having higher levels of male hormones. A woman with less hormonal potential has a slender silhouette.

In search of exceptional athletic performance, some athletes do not hesitate, despite their young age and good health, to take hormones to increase their muscular mass. The use of male hormones is particularly striking in female athletes, whose virile muscular morphology is accompanied by an almost masculine pilosity and temperament.

The International Olympic Committee classifies testosterone as a doping product; its use is prohibited among high-level athletes. The improvement of scores as a result of hormonal doping is an example of the perverse use of hormones.

Cardiac muscle is also sensitive to the effects of testosterone. In animals, testosterone administration increases the quantity of the protein responsible for the heart's contraction (actinomyosin) [3].

In 2013, a study on mice at the Department of Biochemistry, Microbiology, and Immunology of the University of Ottawa, Canada, in partnership with Dasman Diabetes Institute in Kuwait,
showed the stimulation and differentiation of stem cells in cardiac cells due to testosterone by specifying its molecular mechanisms [4].

Bones impregnated with male hormones are solid. Testosterone acts on the skeletal structures by conferring the elasticity necessary for flexibility.

The nervous system and its sensitivity to male hormones are the objects of many studies. Receptors exist in the brain, the nerves, and the spinal cord.

Testosterone ensures memory and supports idea creation. It determines action when its production is sufficient.

There are testosterone molecules in high numbers in the nerve cells responsible for motility and the coordination of movements. The integrity of nerve functions depends, consequently, on the proper secretion of male hormones.

The skin is known for its dependence on male hormones. The prevalence of pilosity in men is a result of androgens, and excessive hair growth among women is a result of the secretion of too many male hormones.

To test the quality of the skin, grip an inch between the thumb and the index finger. Do not exceed one centimeter in thickness. When the fingers slacken, it must regain its shape instantaneously. In contrast, skin that lacks male hormones remains folded for a few moments.

Red blood cell (RBC) counts increase under the influence of male hormones. Women manufacture fewer RBCs than men. In women, the number of RBCs ranges between 4.20 million and 5.4 million in a cubic millimeter of blood.

Many studies show the favorable influence of male hormones on the body's ability to manufacture RBCs.

White blood cells (WBCs) are the guards of immunity. They contain receptors for male hormones. By stimulating the WBCs, male hormones fight directly against infection and cancer.

A study in 2012 even showed that sex hormones stimulate increased telomerase of blood cells and, consequently, their multiplication [5].

The fluidity of the blood depends on the presence of sufficient male hormones stimulating antithrombin, a factor that improves blood flow.

Male hormones make proteins. Testosterone is the hormone of proteins and anabolism—in other words, of the organism's construction.

The liver and the kidneys increase in weight after the administration of male hormones. This is a normal consequence of the presence of recently incorporated proteins, and it acts on functional tissue.

Sugars also depend on male hormones, which act on glycogen and blood glucose.

Fats do not escape the control of androgens. A woman who consults a doctor is almost always aware of her triglyceride and cholesterol levels. Still, she is usually unaware that these levels depend closely on the secretion of male hormones.

In the blood, various fractions represent cholesterol. Those most known by the public are high-density lipoprotein (HDL) cholesterol ("good" cholesterol) and low-density lipoprotein (LDL) cholesterol ("bad" cholesterol). Testosterone favorably influences the metabolism of HDL cholesterol.

Testosterone acts as a regulator of fats in the organism. Cholesterol and triglycerides become pathological because of a disordered state of hormonal secretion. Food plays a part in this disorder, but it is not the only culprit. This is what explains the lack of results in a woman seeking a drop in her levels of blood cholesterol through a draconian regime.

In sum, testosterone acts on all organs and has a role in all bodily functions.

Dihydrotestosterone: The Hormone of Sexual Energy

Good sexual activity is a sign of good health. Here, also, testosterone plays a vital role.

> The sexual organs of women usually function only with **dihydrotestosterone**.

Testosterone is not a sex hormone. It is a hormonal precursor that is transformed locally into the sexually active hormone dihydrotestosterone. How does this occur? Testosterone circulates in the organism, bound to carrying proteins. Those regularly release 2 percent of the total quantity of testosterone. This free testosterone penetrates the organs to do its work there. When it enters the sexual organs, it forms dihydrotestosterone.

One consequently needs proper testosterone secretion for its transformation into dihydrotestosterone, the sexually active derivative.

The surprising thing is that all scientific studies of androgens in postmenopausal women focus only on testosterone. At the same time, dihydrotestosterone is often the solution to a menopausal problem—urinary urgency, for example.

Testosterone Secretion Drops with Age

In the 1970s, a new method of analysis allowed medical professionals to dose hormones with precision. Rosalyn Sussman Yalow developed the radioimmunoassay technique at the Veterans Administration Hospital in the Bronx, New York. This revolutionary development earned Dr. Yalow the Nobel Prize for Medicine in 1977, the second woman ever to win it.

As a woman grows old, she secretes fewer and fewer male hormones, as shown in table 2. The levels of testosterone regularly drop after age twenty-five in women. Studies published in 2004 demonstrated this concept [6,7].

Mean Plasma Concentrations of Testosterone before Menopause	
Age	Results in nanogram/100 mL
20–39	51
30–39	48
40–49	32

Table 2

Based on Guay, Munarriz, Jacobson, Talakoub, Traish, Quirk, Goldstein, and Spark (2004) [6,7].

Regardless of the sophisticated and exciting biochemical studies that are of scientific interest, the interpretation of testosterone levels is easy.

We must consider the correlation of testosterone with the high production of dihydrotestosterone and its high plasma levels in young and healthy women.

With aging, there is not enough testosterone to penetrate the sexual organs (through its transformation in dihydrotestosterone) and other organs. This phenomenon begins the organism's involution and starts the vicious cycle of self-destruction that develops with time and leads to death.

The hormonal Singularity

Epidemiological studies of the hormonal levels in blood give a general idea of what occurs in the population: the decrease of male hormones with aging.

The reduction of the production of testosterone and dihydrotestosterone is unique to each individual. Therefore, the preferable first step is to determine the pool of androgens of an individual. Each woman is unique and has a particular hormonal profile. A complete hormonal profile analyzes the chemical precursors of androgens and their metabolites in the urine. The measurement of the amount of these metabolites present in twenty-four hours makes it possible to specify whether there is a daily hormonal overload or deficiency, making it possible to understand what hormone is needed and how to adjust the therapeutic doses. The measurement of complementary parameters is also useful. All these analyses constitute what I call the *study of the hormonal pool of androgens*.

The reader will find more information about these elements at http://www.georgesdebled.org/pool-androgens-w.htm

This comprehensive analysis is very technical. However, a simple report consisting of assaying testosterone and dihydrotestosterone in the blood is sometimes enough.

3

Treatment with Male Hormones Is an Old Concept

The action of male hormones on the human body has been known for many centuries. Aristotle, for example, noticed the plumpness of eunuchs. At the time of Jesus Christ, the Greeks thought that there was a substance responsible for long life and wondered whether a relationship existed between this and sexual energy.

The effects of a lack of male hormones in animals have also been known for a long time. The capon is a castrated cock. Its sexual characteristics do not develop. Its cockscomb, which is an erectile organ, remains rudimentary. These organs atrophy as a result of a lack of male hormones.

In 1849, Arnold Adolph Berthold showed that the testes secrete a substance able to act remotely on the voice, the plumage, and the cockscomb of capons.

Biologists have gradually elucidated the chemical structures of sex hormones, facilitating the ability to make synthetics. In 1931, Adolf Butenandt found fifteen milligrams of androsterone in seventeen thousand liters of male urine, isolated in the form of crystals [1]. This substance has an androgenic effect. A few years later, researchers clarified the chemical structure of androsterone as that of testosterone, which is the male hormone itself.

In 1935, Léopold Ruzicka developed the artificial synthesis of testosterone. This synthetic hormone is not very soluble. The duration of its action is short. Thus, this substance is not appropriate for hormonal treatment. In 1939, Butenandt and Ruzicka obtained the Nobel Prize in chemistry for their discoveries.

In 1937, researchers modified the testosterone molecule. They made an androgenic derivative that is soluble in oils: testosterone propionate. Injected intramuscularly, it reabsorbs slowly. From this time, doctors immediately began using this hormone, of which they knew the biological properties.

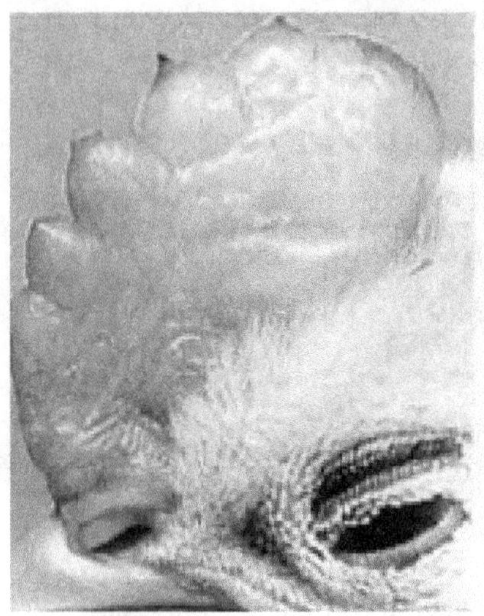

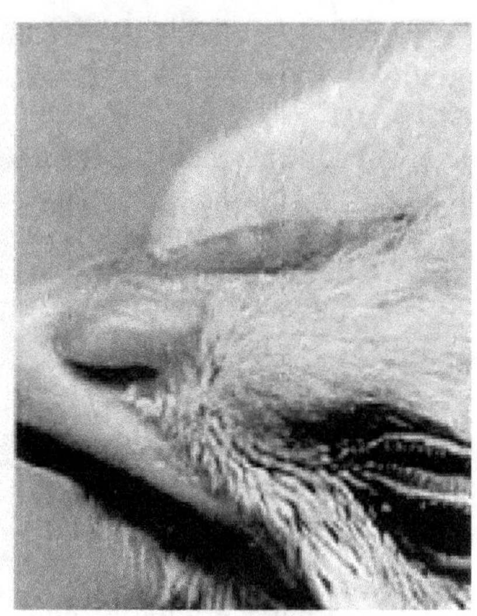

Fig 1.

A. Cockscomb with hormones. B. Cockscomb in castrated cock.

On the right (B): small castrated cock. The cockscomb, which is an erectile body, is not developed (Shering document).

On the left (A): the same cock treated with mesterolone; the cockscomb develops and is erectile (Shering document).

The woman's clitoris is also erectile and atrophies in the absence of dihydrotestosterone; the potent sex hormone usually made daily in sufficient quantity in women.

As early as 1938, doctors undertook therapy with testosterone in women afflicted with various gynecological and sexual disorders [2,3].

In 1941, Berlind noted the beneficial effects of androgens in ameliorating various gynecological disorders in 106 women. Numerous symptoms improved after methyltestosterone treatment [4]. But we know today that methyltestosterone has a toxic effect on the liver.

Androgens are synthesized in the female and are the precursors of estrogen biosynthesis. It has been known since 1941 that if there is no testosterone, there are no female hormones [5].

Androgenic disease of menopause starts with a failure to produce adequate dihydrotestosterone. There was no specific treatment for menopausal disease before the late 1960s when mesterolone arrived on the market. Mesterolone is a mostly safe drug that mimics dihydrotestosterone (and testosterone).

In 1968, Nicholas Bruchovsky and Jean D. Wilson from Texas University, Dallas, discovered the conversion of testosterone to dihydrotestosterone in the rat prostate [6]. That same year, K. M. Anderson and Shutsung Liao from the University of Chicago found specific receptors for dihydrotestosterone in the nuclei of prostate cells of rats [7]. Despite those discoveries, it is surprising that mesterolone is unknown in the United States. Therefore, in the United States, it is impossible to replace the missing hormone to treat the first stages of androgenic menopausal disease, which is one of the early stages of aging. Surprisingly, mesterolone is available worldwide—in Canada, Brazil, Mexico, the United Kingdom, China, Asia, and the European Union. My studies with mesterolone in women, which began in 1998 and have continued to the present day, have shown no side effects. It is all the more surprising that methyltestosterone, a toxic hormone, is available in the United States.

In the United States, then, the problem seems to be that it is difficult to treat a disease whose existence is unknown with a drug that is not available. In contrast, it should be a blockbuster drug for the pharmaceutical industry.

The diagnosis of androgenic menopausal disease did not exist before 1974, the year when radioimmunoassays (RIAs) became available in daily medical practice. Radioimmunological analyses that determined the proportion of dihydrotestosterone, testosterone, and their metabolites were consequently realizable.

Despite the clinical use of testosterone in women throughout much of the twentieth century, contemporary testosterone therapy in women is hotly debated, misunderstood, and often misrepresented in the medical community.

In 2006, the Canadian Consensus Conference on Menopause concluded that more studies about testosterone in women were necessary, with the concept of androgen insufficiency remaining imprecise [8]. This consensus ignored *androgenic disease of menopause*, which is a different concept than "menopause." The word *dihydrotestosterone* was not used once in the 112 pages of conclusions of this consensus.

Since 1974, I have prescribed male hormone replacement therapy (HRT) to men deprived of hormones [9–32]. These treatments invariably restore physical ability, mental ability, and sexual activity and are described in *Ageless Man*, published in 2017.

At that time, numerous women consulted my urological service for urinary problems that were not addressed at practices anywhere in my country, mainly, the urgency to urinate without the presence of infection, sometimes leading to urinary incontinence.

I realized immediately that the urinary symptoms in women were like those of young men having prostate atrophy. That is, with a posterior urethra like the female urethra, the bladder outlet was a hormonal target that needed male hormones (dihydrotestosterone) to open and close normally.

Seeing the surprisingly good results of this potent HRT in male urinary problems, their wives asked to follow a treatment that could give similar good results. Women with urinary symptoms were the first of my patients who were interested in finding a hormonal solution to their urinary problems.

At the time, conventional HRT for women posed safety problems, as we will see later.

I started to study the question in 1998. Because young and healthy women physiologically produce more male hormones every day than female hormones, I simply wondered what this normal or pathological production could be and what the consequences of a possible lack of androgens might be.

The results of my study were immediate. Women producing fewer male hormones had disorders similar to those of men with disruptions in male hormones. My male patients were suffering from urinary problems and andropause disease—*androgenic disease of andropause*. So, I started to prescribe specific treatments to replace the missing male hormones with mesterolone in aging women, with impressive results.

The concept of *menopausal disease* or *androgenic disease of menopause* was presented for the first time before a meeting of doctors in October 2015 at the Spanish Society of Anti-Aging Medicine and Longevity (SEMAL) Congress in Madrid and published in *Approaches to Aging Control* in October 2015 [29].

4

A Vigorous Longevity beyond Eighty Years

Women and men constitute the most complex living structures. Their molecular combinations are the most developed, and they have the most elaborate brain structure among living things. Today, the purely animal cerebral evolution of human beings has arrived at its end. The development has reached a critical stage: the spiritual transformation of humankind. This planetary phenomenon, this change without precedent in human history, is in a latent state in each one of us. The great adventure has already started. Gradually, human beings release themselves from the constraints of animalism.

We remember test-tube babies—that is all it took to dissociate human reproduction from the act of coupling. Genetic progress will make it possible to avoid nonviable congenital anomalies. Human reproduction will one day be without risk, both for children and mothers. The first stages of life are already scientifically reproducible, so we should be astonished by the lack of interest that surrounds the last steps.

A woman lives today according to a reverse mode that constitutes a dead-end for the future of humanity. From birth to the beginning of menopausal disease—the androgenic disease of menopause—she generally lives in good health for forty years, the lifetime of a woman in the Middle Ages.

The last forty years of a woman's life is senescence or moving toward decline and death. When, after forty, sometimes even before, sexual, and reproductive regression become effective, it announces the arrival of successive physical and psychic degradations. Therefore, in the absence of hormonal prevention of aging and despite the remedies of traditional medicine, no reasonable solution can be found. With the giant deficit in terms of health insurance, and the lack of affordable health care, the solution for this crucial economic problem depends primarily on a scientific, biological approach. To age in good health is inexpensive.

Women beyond forty are prone to a decrease in sexual activity, with accompanying slowness of movement and mentality.

During the second half of their existence, women degenerate. This degradation is regarded as impossible to stop. There is a gigantic hole in our knowledge because we are unaware of all the causes of aging, whose consequences, in contrast, are well indexed and treated.

Understanding sexual regression and the degradation that follows is the right approach toward senescence because it is possible to mitigate its effects with the use of mesterolone. But this is addressed only to the woman who reflects on herself, for the excellent reason that she must understand and take part in her treatment.

Fifty thousand years ago, the woman's morphology changed little. The essential changes concentrated on the human brain. This phenomenon became more and more complex, becoming the dominating factor. Socialization of minds exists. Minds worldwide have connected, thanks to the deployment of communication resources. When an event occurs, it is the entire planet that reacts. Tensions in the world are a striking example. This phenomenon of brains' interconnection causes a new right, that of access to information. But not all are in the same boat.

There are tribes in existence today that live in the age of fire. Certain natives of tropical areas have a life expectancy of approximately twenty years. Whole populations still live according to the medieval mode and have a considerably reduced life expectancy. In Europe, in endangered industrial sites, communities still live at the beginning of the twentieth century. In modern cities, one sees men and women who are defined primarily as consumers.

From the forest, via fields and cities, the woman became a consumer unparalleled, and nothing is off-limits anymore. Obsessed with having, she overlooked the road to the highest form of life: being.

But the progressive woman is deep within. It is enough to boost her with information. She will then be able to understand and treat her aging.

Failing this, what do we do? Despite the massive deployment of technological means, average longevity does not exceed eighty years, and after forty years, a woman slows down sexually, physically, and mentally. She is unaware that she doesn't secrete enough male hormones. In addition to this lack of knowledge, the disastrous effects of overeating, and the total lack of muscular exercise are common.

After forty, it is initially necessary to reflect and decide to live, thanks to hormonal therapy with androgens, with a controlled food diet and exercise. Women who see their symptoms disappear with hormonal treatment become able to diagnose their recovery from menopausal disease by examining other untreated women, reflections of what they were before. The woman with menopausal syndrome shows typical characteristics. Most obvious is the lack of brightness. Conversely, the general health condition of women treated with mesterolone is surprising.

Birth and death are natural phenomena that belong to the realm of metaphysics. Between these two poles, there is life. It is essential to know it best, to overcome physical obstacles, and to use its spiritual potential as much as possible. Here, industrial medicine, birthed from scientific medicine, missed the mark. Indeed, medicine has the aim of saving and reestablishing health, which is not only an absence of disease or infirmity but also a state of mental and social well-being. However, the medicine that has developed for forty years, according to the characteristics of industrial civilization, is only able to eliminate disease and infirmity, being unaware of the state of mental and social well-being.

Does the reader know that the price of highly sophisticated apparatuses is fixed not by their manufacturing costs and a reasonable profit but by the number of patients likely to use them and according to refunding by Social Security offices? Is wanting to escape from the natural phenomenon of death quite reasonable? Too many patients die today encumbered by machinery, even when they have reached eighty years, the limit of longevity in the industrial era. Frustrating deaths. Unworthy deaths.

The most frequent diseases today are those of discomfort, whose causes are not very visible. They require a *comprehensive approach* to the individual, which is well understood by experts of medicine. Such methods often contribute to the reestablishment of the physical and mental well-being, essential components of health, and are not as parallel as some would like to make-believe.

Causes of aging are the primary source of discomfort. They must be the subject of individual attention. What do we note? Before forty, women are generally in good health, and they have good sexual activity. Menopause marks the end of the reproductive program. Gradually, aging diseases occur—osteoarthritis, arteriosclerosis, obesity, cataracts, and skin, nail, and hair disorders. Cerebral activity is disturbed, and disorders of the memory appear. Migraines, gloomy moods, lack of dynamism, pusillanimity, unhappiness, and depression, up to that point unknown, make their appearance. These symptoms are often signs of menopausal disease.

To treat menopausal disease—the androgenic condition of menopause—means to decrease, if not eliminate, aging diseases so that women beyond age forty will remain in good health.

With proper treatment, mature human beings will no longer know the inexorable decrepitude that leads to death at around age eighty. Women and men of fifty, sixty, and seventy years will have the aspects of their forties and be in good health. The older woman of sixty chronological years will be biologically forty after replacing her defective parameters for twenty years.

This difference between the chronological age and the biological age currently exists. For example, embryos are preserved in liquid nitrogen at a low temperature. When implanted in the mother, an embryo gives rise to a human being. An embryo frozen for two months results in a child whose chronological age is eleven months and whose biological age is nine months. Thus, an old embryo of several consecutive years would give rise to a being whose biological age would be only nine months.

For the first time, humans have started to understand the mechanisms that govern the beginning and the end of their terrestrial existence. Today, it is necessary to study aging's causes. The task is immense. Comprehension of the mechanisms of aging will allow the full use of human resources, from birth to death. Women treated with mesterolone will reach their potential longevity. They will be ageless women.

Centenaries are the expression of the potential of longevity. But when they are not treated, they do no longer run like rabbits. With individually designed hormonal treatment, one can imagine that the human being can potentially live to around 120 years old, perhaps more. The key is to get there in good health; if not, it is useless.

Specific hormones open the door to this possibility. Centenaries will not live isolated in their rooms and without activity. We will finally be able to "die of life." Experiments show that the blood levels of male hormones are high in older adults who are still ripe and active. These are precisely the women who could become centenaries without HRT.

Older women treated correctly with mesterolone are simply in the same situation as young women whose ovaries secrete male hormones naturally and who enjoy exceptional health. If one stops the treatment of an older woman enjoying good health thanks to correct replacement by mesterolone, she will invariably degrade again, physically, mentally, and sexually.

The treatment and prevention of aging diseases will increase the average longevity of a population. We will see, in twenty years, septuagenarians whose biological age will be fifty years. Conscious of their menopausal disease—their androgenic disease of menopause—they will have been treated. In a few decades, centenaries will be in good health thanks to the right hormonal treatment, and nobody can say today what the age limit will be.

Part II

Genital Aging

5

Aging of Women's Masculine Genitalia

The masculine genitalia of women are as follows:

- The clitoris and its foreskin (the male counterparts are the penis and prepuce)
- The labia majora (homologs of the scrotum in humans)
- The bladder neck (the posterior muscular segment of the urethra; homologous to the prostatic musculature in humans)

These organs are targets for dihydrotestosterone, the sex hormone.

Aging of Sexual Organs

The masculine genitalia of women atrophy after menopause. There is progressive atrophy of the clitoris and labia majora. This can result in pain during penetration and an absence of libido. Troubles of micturition are frequent.

Origin of Androgen Production in Women

Androgens are produced daily in the ovaries, adrenals, and peripheral tissues, constituting the *total androgen production.* With aging, the daily androgen output varies in those three pathways. When the ovaries' production of androgens decreases for one reason or another (e.g., aging, removal of the ovaries, androgenic disease of menopause), the total pool of androgens is diminished.

When the total daily production is sufficient, they are no symptoms of androgen deficiency.

Women do not begin to suffer from androgen deficiency at the same age. When their remaining total secretion of androgens is ample enough—calculated by adding the production of the ovaries, adrenal glands, and dihydrotestosterone—they have no symptoms of androgen deficiency.

Therefore, to make a correct diagnosis and establish an effective treatment plan, the global pool of androgens must always be specified by analyzing the production chains and metabolic chains.

It is somewhat surprising to note that the scientific studies whose characteristics correspond to the standards recognized by high-level journals do not mention the daily production of androgens in general, and even fewer mention dihydrotestosterone specifically.

Regular Production of Testosterone during the Normal Menstrual Cycle

Testosterone and Estradiol Production in Micrograms/Day during the Normal Menstrual Cycle [1]		
	Estradiol	Testosterone
Proliferative phase	40	200
Secretory phase	200	200

Table 3

According to Baulieu and Kelly [1].

Before menopause, a normal woman produces 5-fold more testosterone than estradiol each day in the proliferative phase and the same quantity in the secretory phase [1], as shown in table 3.

In healthy women, plasma dihydrotestosterone represents almost 50 percent of testosterone levels, as shown in table 4.

The Woman before Menopause: Plasma Hormonal Concentrations in Nanograms/100 mL [1] *	
Testosterone	57 ± 19 ng/100 mL
Dihydrotestosterone	**27 ± 6 ng/100 mL**

Table 4

* The standards depend on the methods of analysis. That is why we must always refer to the same laboratory.

In healthy women, the plasma level of testosterone is still higher than that of estradiol.

Testosterone–Dihydrotestosterone–Estradiol Plasma Levels in Picograms/100 mL during the Normal Menstrual Cycle (Mean Levels) [1]			
	Estradiol	Testosterone	Dihydrotestosterone
Proliferative phase	6,000	57,000	27,000
Secretory phase	20,000	57,000	27,000

Table 5

In women, the concentration of testosterone in plasma is always higher than the estradiol concentration. The plasma concentration of testosterone is approximately tenfold the level of estradiol during the proliferative phase and nearly threefold the level of estradiol during the secretory period. The testosterone secretion increases during ovulation (as measured by direct radioimmunoassay [RIA]) in the healthy menstrual cycle [2]. The production of dihydrotestosterone in young and healthy women is essential—more than fourfold the level of estradiol during the proliferative phase and approximately 1.5-fold the level of estradiol during the secretory period (table 5).

Testosterone Secretion Regularly Decreases from the Age of Twenty in Women

The expected testosterone concentration in the blood of a woman of age forty would be about half that of a woman of age twenty-one [3]. After menopause, the decreases in the secretion of testosterone and dihydrotestosterone are significant and can be quite impressive, as shown in the following table (note that these parameters have been known for more than thirty years):

The Woman, before and after Menopause [1]: Plasma Hormonal Concentrations in Nanograms (ng)/100 mL		
	Before Menopause	After Menopause
Testosterone	57 ± 19 ng/100 mL	**15 – 5 ng/100 mL**
Dihydrotestosterone	27 ± 6 ng/100 mL	**8 – 5 ng/ 100 mL**

Table 6

Apart from reproductive engineering, which mainly involves the female hormones estradiol and progesterone, the well-being of women depends, before and after menopause, on the proper secretion of testosterone and dihydrotestosterone before menopause and their replacement after menopause.

Androstanediol glucuronide is a metabolite of dihydrotestosterone. Its level in the blood gives an idea about the available dihydrotestosterone. Low androstanediol glucuronide signifies low dihydrotestosterone in the plasma.

The effects of excess of testosterone and dihydrotestosterone on the masculine genitalia of women are well known. An excess of dihydrotestosterone results in different degrees of virilization (for more information, see http://www.georgesdebled.org/masculine%20genitalia.htm).

Androstanediol Glucuronide: Plasma Hormonal Concentrations in Nanograms (ng)/mL [1]		
	Before Menopause	After Menopause
Androstanediol glucuronide	± 5.4 ng/mL	**± 0.5 ng/mL**

Table 7

A detailed biological study is sometimes necessary to consider the hormonal parameters.

Two significant pathologies are the consequence of a lack of dihydrotestosterone:

- Bladder neck sclerosis and micturition problems
- Vaginal dryness

Bladder Neck Sclerosis and Inflammation

As a urologist, I have experience with bladder neck sclerosis (and its endoscopic surgery) in women dating back to 1971. In 1998, I discovered the role of dihydrotestosterone in the female bladder neck and the beneficial effect of mesterolone on this pathology. No description of the impact of mesterolone on the bladder neck existed in the world literature until the publication of *The Menopausal Disease* in October 2015 [4].

Sclerosis of bladder neck in menopause produces the following:

- Chronic cystitis
- Incontinence
- Urgency to urinate

The bladder neck is a muscular structure. Its function is to open during micturition. This structure is sensitive to male hormones, which ensure its integrity. The bladder neck musculature atrophies in the absence of dihydrotestosterone, and fibrous tissue replaces it. Mesterolone is the right treatment. One can even wonder whether the "traditional" medications of hormonal replacement therapy (HRT) worsen bladder neck fibrosis. Treatment with mesterolone prevents the atrophy of the bladder neck musculature among women deprived of dihydrotestosterone. The results are often spectacular.

Urethra and Bladder Neck in Women

The urethra comprises three parts of approximately the same length (one centimeter in the adult woman):

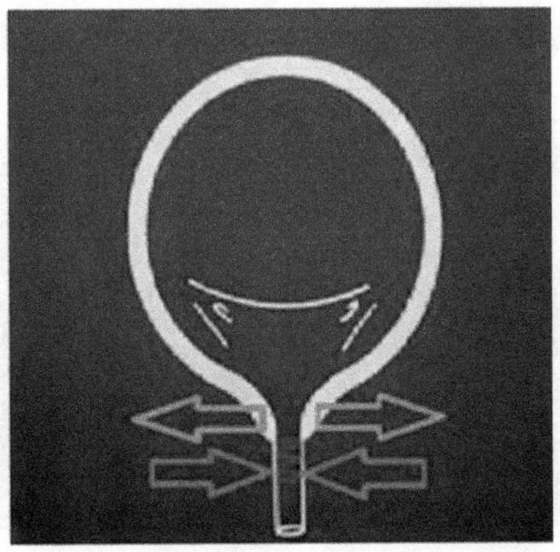

Fig. 2
The function of the bladder neck.

- The inner part is formed by fibromuscular tissue in continuity with the fibromuscular tissue of the bladder (bladder neck).
- The sphincter constitutes the medium part.
- The external section is a conduit.

Fibrosis of the Bladder Neck in Women

Fibrosis of the bladder neck can be congenital, but a significant number of cases develop during life. During opening (light grey arrows in the figure 2), the bladder neck does not work well, and its maximum diameter is often less than one centimeter. There is no acute urinary system infection, yet women complain of symptoms. Doctors often consider these women as "psychotic." The figures 3 to 5 show the effect of sclerosis on the opening from the bladder neck.

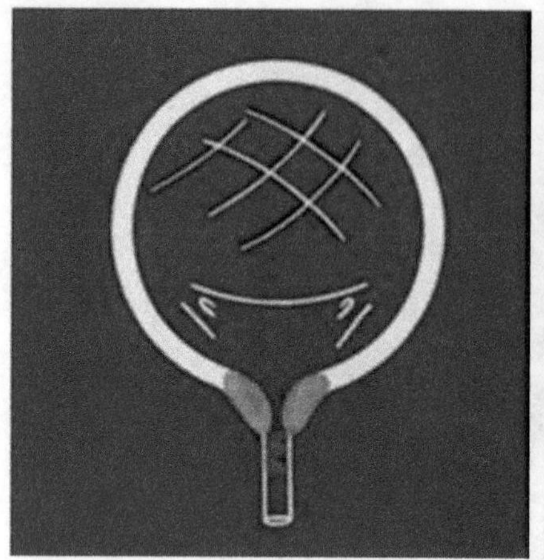

Fig. 3
Sclerosis of the bladder neck produces a narrowing of the posterior urethra.

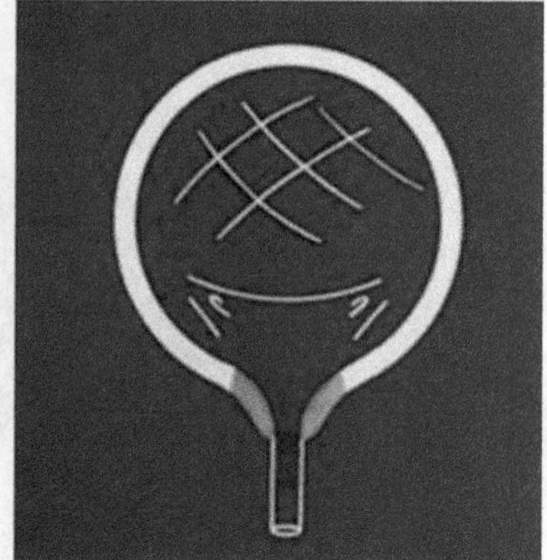

Fig. 4
Sclerosis of the bladder neck without narrowing of posterior urethra.

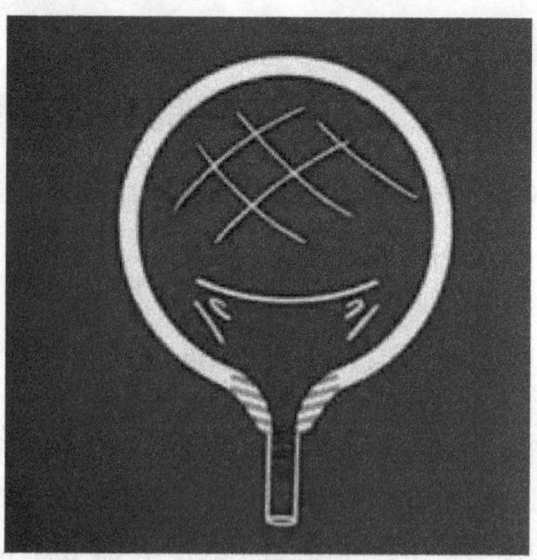

Fig. 5

Moderate sclerosis of the bladder neck without reduction of the posterior urethra.

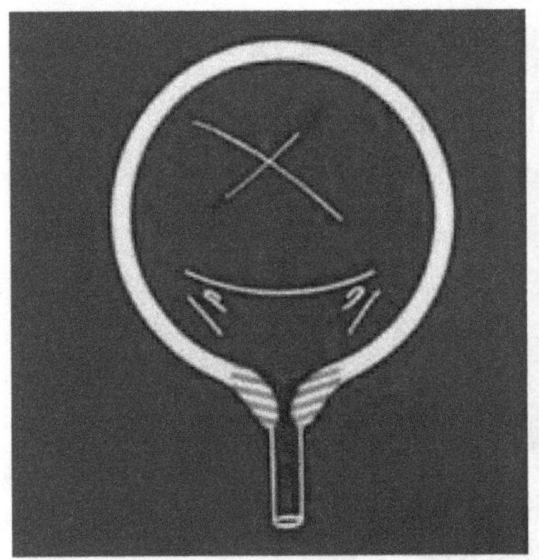

Fig. 6

Sclerosis of bladder neck and congestion.

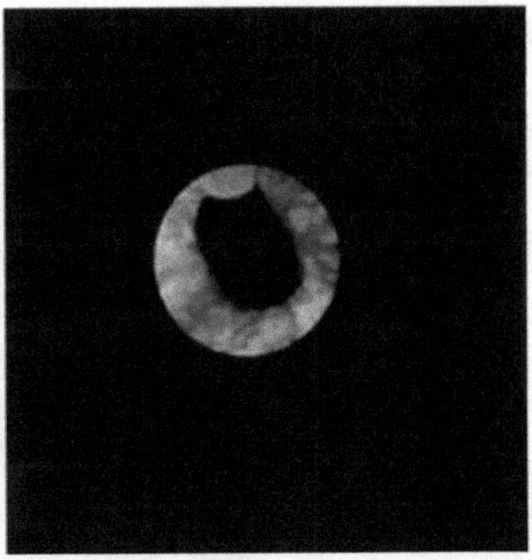

Fig. 7

Endoscopy: Sclerosis of bladder neck and congestion.

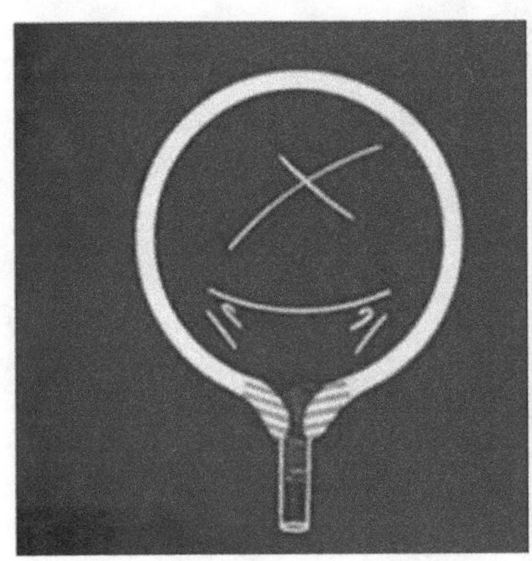

Fig. 8

Sclerosis of the bladder neck. Inflammation and inflammatory polyps.

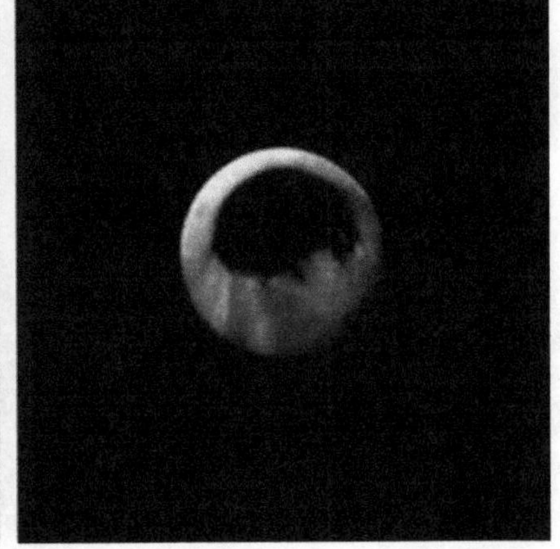

Fig. 9

Endoscopy: Sclerosis of the bladder neck. Inflammation and inflammatory polyps.

Pathology of Bladder Neck Sclerosis in Women

The histological sections show healthy, typical bladder neck (fig.10) structures and fibrosis of the bladder neck (fig.11).

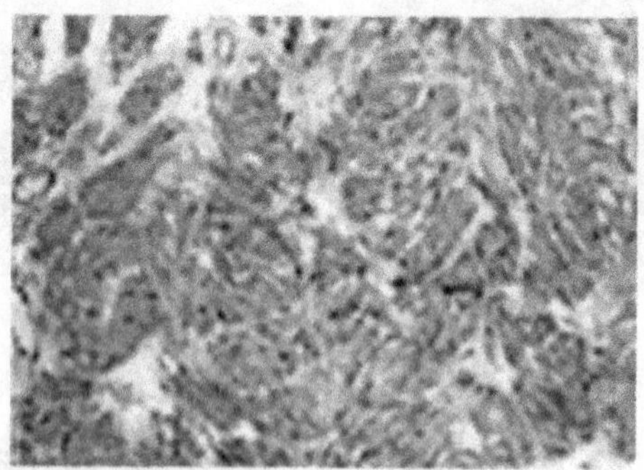

Fig. 10
Healthy musculature of the bladder neck.

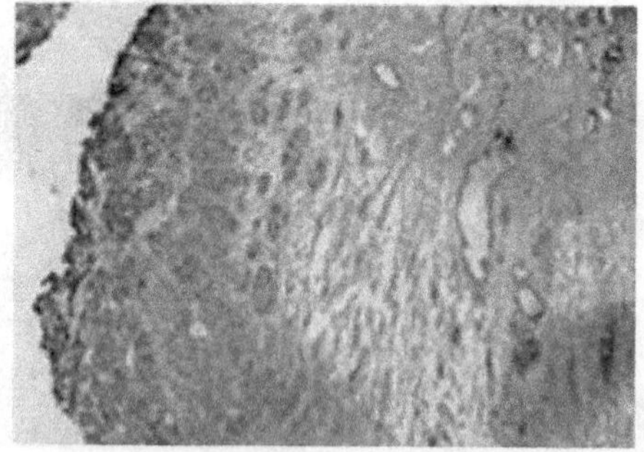

Fig. 11
Sclerosis of the bladder neck in women.

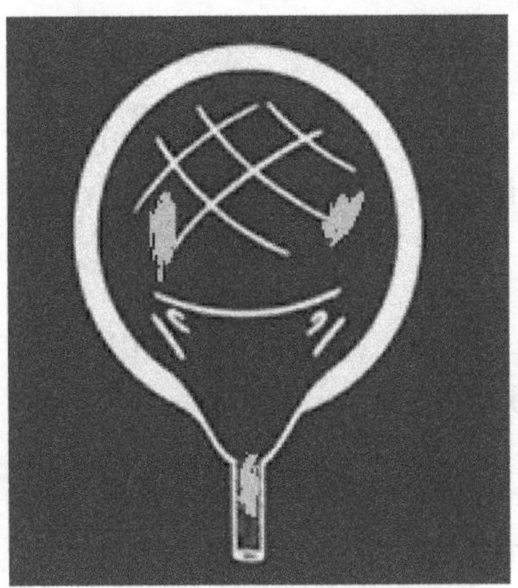

Fig. 12
Immediately after bladder neck resection of fibrous tissue, inflammation may remain in the bladder wall or anterior urethra (in light grey).

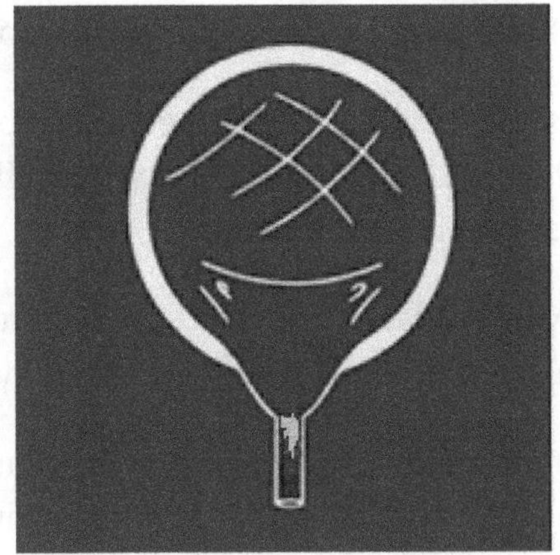

Fig. 13
Immediately after bladder neck resection of fibrous tissue, inflammation may remain in the anterior urethra (in light grey).

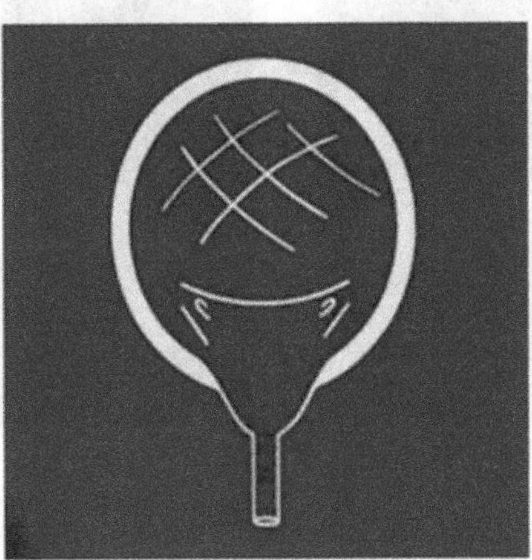

Fig. 14
After bladder neck resection of fibrous tissue, inflammation generally disappears within three months.

Bladder Neck Resection for Fibrosis in Women

Before bladder neck resection of fibrous tissue, when the opening of the bladder neck does not work well, its maximum diameter is often less than one centimeter.

After bladder neck resection of fibrous tissue, the opening of the bladder neck diameter enlarges to two to three centimeters.

In the patient case shown in the figures 15 and 16, the opening after bladder neck resection was five centimeters.

Evolution of Lower Urinary Tract Infection after Removal of Bladder Neck Sclerosis in Women

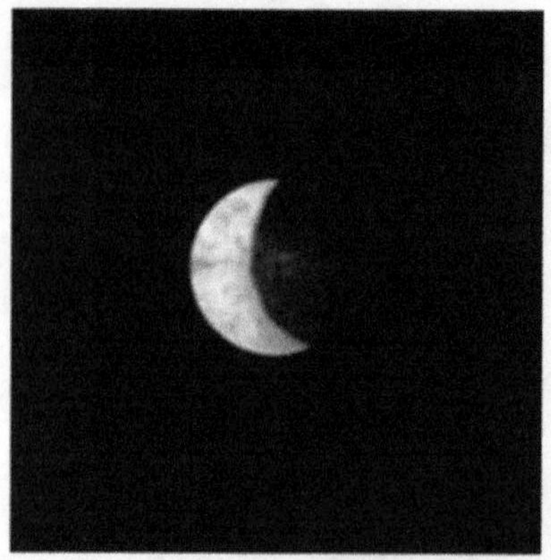

Fig. 15
Bladder neck after resection of fibrous tissue: right side.

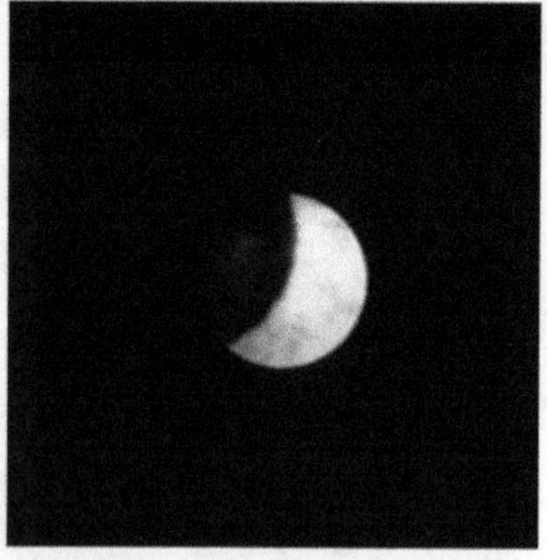

Fig. 16
Bladder neck after resection of fibrous tissue: left side.

- Immediately after bladder neck resection of fibrous tissue, inflammation may remain in the bladder wall or anterior urethra.

- Immediately after bladder neck resection of fibrous tissue, inflammation may remain in the anterior urethra.

- After bladder neck resection of fibrous tissue, inflammation generally disappears entirely within three months.

Mechanical Consequences of Bladder Neck Sclerosis

Bladder neck fibrosis provokes hypertrophy of the bladder musculature or, later, a weak bladder musculature. Poor opening of the bladder neck leads to secondary narrowing of the terminal ureter, hypertension in the upper urinary tract, and reduced functioning of the kidneys—in summary: the destruction of the urinary tract [5] (see chapter 22).

Incidence of Deficiency of Androgens in the Female Bladder Neck

Mesterolone treatment spectacularly cured a 70-year-old woman with a lack of androgens. Her bladder neck was congestive, with abnormal sensitivity. This woman's urologist had proposed an endoscopic surgery, which was postponed thanks to mesterolone treatment. This woman has been free of symptoms since 2003. If sclerosis and congestion of the bladder neck are not too severe, mesterolone can normalize urination in women. However, sclerosis sometimes requires endoscopic removal of the pathological tissue, followed by mesterolone preventive treatment to prevent the recurrence of congestion and sclerosis.

I presented this topic at the Spanish Society of Anti-Aging Medicine and Longevity (SEMAL) Congress in October 2015 in Madrid [4]. Since then, family doctors have been prescribing mesterolone treatment for their female patients with micturition troubles. Diagnosis and treatment are cheap and straightforward. The results are impressive.

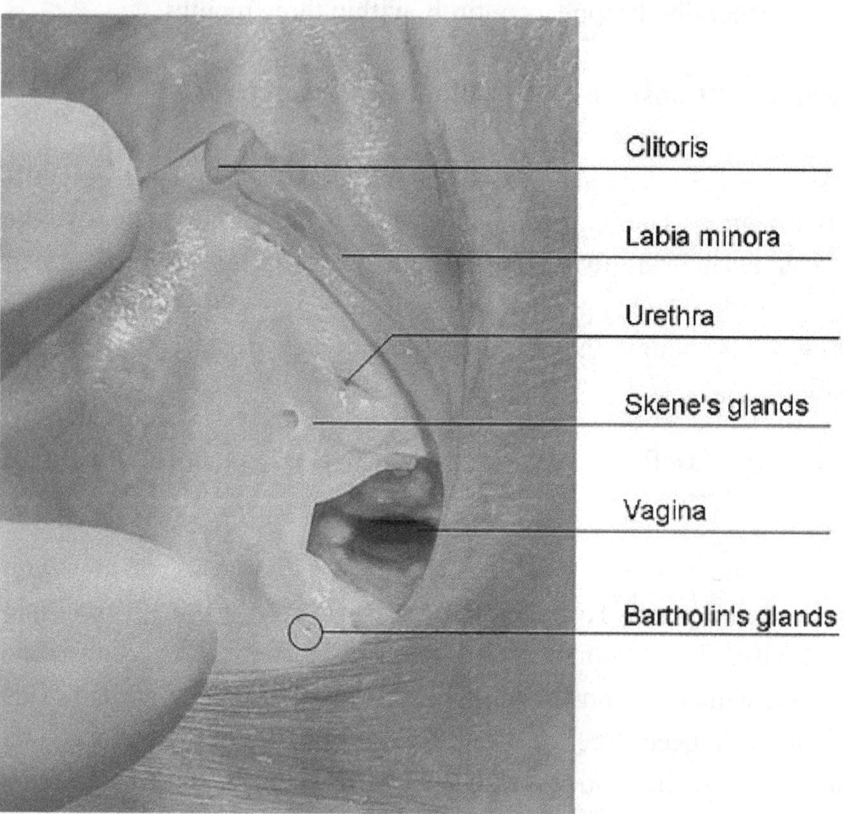

Fig. 17
From Nicholasolan at English Wikipedia.

Vaginal Dryness

Vaginal dryness does not have only a vaginal cause. It comes from a lack of lubrication from the masculine genital glands located at the entrance of the vagina, at the vulva.

Medical treatment is specific to dihydrotestosterone and *not with female hormones*. A lack of secretions from the masculine genital glands provokes vaginal dryness during intercourse. Those glands are situated at the entry of the vagina, as shown in the figure 17.

Bartholin's glands are located on each side of the posterior part of the lower vaginal opening (at the junction of the middle third and posterior third of the vulva), in the thickness of the labia majora.

These two glands are small until puberty. During the period of genital activity, they measure ten to fifteen millimeters in length, eight millimeters in height, and five millimeters in thickness. They are homologous to the Cowper's glands in men that contribute to the ejaculate. Under the influence of sexual arousal and the male hormone dihydrotestosterone, these glands secrete the "love juice," a liquid that lubricates the vulva and vagina. Bartholin's glands do not work until puberty. They regress and stop working after menopause.

Skene's glands are located on the anterior wall of the vagina, around the lower end of the urethra. Their involvement in lubrication is minimal, and it is the two Bartholin's glands that deliver—by two small orifices located in the furrow separating the hymen and the labia minor—a small quantity of this lubricating liquid. The volume of this lubrication is variable and can persist after intercourse.

Bartholin's glands and Skene's glands are lubricating glands that depend on the male hormone dihydrotestosterone. At the time of menopause, they are no longer stimulated by hormones because these hormones are no longer produced by the ovaries (testosterone) and in masculine glands (dihydrotestosterone), creating a collateral inconvenience: vaginal dryness.

Vaginal Receptors to Androgens

The vagina has many receptors that need androgens to be stimulated [6]. With HRT treatment, female hormones will worsen the vaginal dryness by inhibiting what remains of androgen production.

6

Aging of the Reproductive Organs

Reproductive Organs

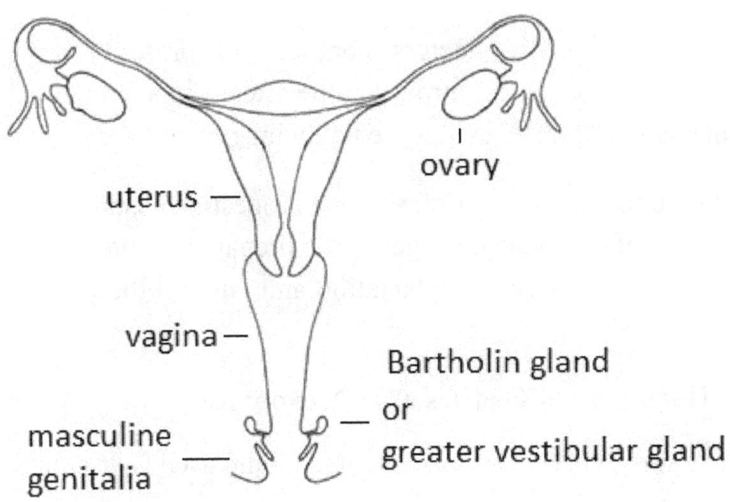

Fig. 18

This diagram (frontal section) shows the female reproductive system and masculine genitalia.

After the original drawing by Eric Walravens.

The female genitals of women are the organs for human reproduction. This function begins with puberty and finishes with menopause, which appears around fifty years of age. The little girls born today will be able to live a hundred years and more. They will not be fertile for more than approximately thirty-five years after the age of fifteen. After this time, they will no longer be capable of human reproduction.

The main female reproductive organs are the ovaries, fallopian tubes, uterus, and vagina. The reproductive apparatus of a woman depends primarily on two ovarian hormones: estradiol and progesterone. The cycles of production of these hormones begin with puberty and finish at the time of menopause.

One can wonder why doctors continue to prescribe progestin hormones, estrogens, or progesterone after menopause because pregnancy is impossible; ovules are not being produced.

According to the dictionary definition, a progestin substance supports the processes of pregnancy. Progesterone prepares the uterine mucous membrane for the ovule's implantation and ensures the pregnancy's maintenance.

Female Hormones of Ovaries after Menopause

These analyses depend on the dosing technique used [1] (table 8).

To speak about "treatment of menopause in general" begs the question of the cessation of menstruation and ovulation not being a disease.

Consequently, treatment of "menopause" with estrogen or progesterone is generally prescribed at random and can even have adverse effects.

Vaginal Atrophy

Vaginal atrophy (atrophic vaginitis) is the thinning of the vaginal walls.

Vaginal atrophy commonly occurs after menopause. For many women, vaginal atrophy makes the sexual act painful. Urinary disorders often accompany this atrophy.

The Woman after Menopause: Estradiol Plasma Hormone Concentrations [1]		
	Average values ± SD pg./mL	Extreme values pg./mL
GCMS*	5.6 ± 3.8	1-25
Direct methods	6.4 ± 5.4	1.4-36
Indirect methods	9.4 ± 6.3	1.5-45.2

Table 8

Atrophy of the vaginal walls is linked with a lack of estriol. This weak estrogen comes from the transformation of estradiol, which is not produced after menopause.

The shortage of androgens produces dryness, inflammation, and sclerosis of the vulva. There is then a lack of lubrication from the male genital glands at the entrance of the vagina at the vulva (see discussion in the previous chapter). This results in an abnormal sensitivity during intercourse, with the clitoris also becoming atrophied and painful. In this case, a lack of dihydrotestosterone—the masculine hormone—is responsible for the pain during sexual acts. The use of estrogen, regardless of the type used, is thus a mistake, mainly because the

* Gas chromatography–mass spectrometry.

hormonal diagnosis is simple and made by measuring testosterone and dihydrotestosterone in the blood.

Genitourinary Syndrome of Menopause

In May 2013, the International Society for the Study of Women's Sexual Health and the North American Menopause Society cosponsored a terminology consensus conference on vaginal atrophy. Experts agreed on a more precise definition for *atrophic vaginitis* and its concomitant urinary symptoms. The adopted term is *genitourinary syndrome of menopause* (GSM) [2].

But for many suffering women and their doctors, "GSM" remains a mystery. The competent medical approach is to recognize that two pathologies can be concomitant. Now, what will be the right treatment?

The lack of secretion of dihydrotestosterone (see the previous discussion) provokes urinary disorders. The vagina contains many androgen receptors, and androgen administration increases the androgen-receptor expression in both the mucosa and stroma of the human vagina.

GSM is a concept that mixes the urinary symptoms and the genital symptoms of a disease. *Androgenic disease of menopause* [3] has a specific, safe, and cheap treatment: mesterolone. It is probably the cornerstone treatment of GSM (chapter 31).

7

Premature Genital Aging

Around age twenty-five, the concentration of testosterone (and also dihydrotestosterone) in the blood is at its maximum, achieving the construction of the entire body. Then those secretions begin to decrease progressively. The expected testosterone concentration in the blood of a woman of age forty would be about half that of a woman of age twenty-one. After forty, the decrease continues and produces diseases of aging that are the consequences of weak androgen production.

Birth Control Pills

The use of the contraceptive pill aggravates the decrease in the production of male hormones and thus accelerates the aging of the entire structure of the body (see part III). Contraceptive pills have been used by hundreds of millions of women throughout the world and are used by one in four women under age forty-five in the United States.

Do Birth Control Pills Work?

Oral contraceptives inhibit ovulation by suppressing the stimulating production of hypophysis hormones (follicle-stimulating hormone [FSH] and luteinizing hormone [LH]) that control ovulation. Therefore, the secretion of all ovarian steroids is also suppressed, including estrogens, progesterone, and *testosterone, which is necessary to produce dihydrotestosterone, the real sex hormone.*

Common Side Effects of Birth Control Pills

Many women taking contraceptive pills are depressed, have urination problems, and experience decreased libido. Dihydrotestosterone deficiency in women provokes urinary problems and sex problems. Both of these can be solved by mesterolone administration [1].

Regarding the lack of libido or lack of female desire, it is surprising to note that most medical studies focus on the influence of testosterone in women. However, this hormone has no sexual action by itself (see chapter 2).

Birth Control Chart from the FDA

The US Food and Drug Administration (FDA) describes the available methods of contraception and the failure rate of each technique.

According to the FDA:

> If you do not want to get pregnant, there are many birth controls options to choose; no one product is best for everyone. Some methods are more effective than others at preventing pregnancy. Check the pregnancy rates on this chart to get an idea of how effective the product is at preventing pregnancy. The pregnancy rates tell you the number of pregnancies expected per 100 women during the first year of typical use. Typical use shows how effective the different methods are during actual use (including sometimes using a method in a way that is not correct or not consistent). The only sure way to avoid pregnancy is not to have any sexual contact. Talk to your healthcare provider about the best method for you.

According to the contraceptive method used, women may experience the following side effects:

- Irregular bleeding
- No menstruation (amenorrhea)
- Menstrual changes
- Spotting or bleeding between menstrual periods
- Headache
- Mood changes or depressed mood
- Weight gain
- Abdominal or pelvic pain, stomach pain, nausea
- Breast sensitivity
- Skin irritation, allergic reactions, acne
- Urinary infection

Birth control methods that use patches, implants, pills, injections, or intrauterine devices, including estrogen with or without progestin, can result in decreased production of male hormones.

Breast Cancer Risk

Breast cancer is number-one cancer in women, both in the developed and the developing world. The incidence of breast cancer is increasing in the developing world as a result of an increase in life expectancy.

As noted by the International Agency for Research on Cancer (IARC), several risk factors for breast cancer are well documented. Those who use oral contraceptives or hormone replacement therapy (HRT) are at higher risk than non-users. *However, for most women presenting with breast cancer, it is not possible to identify specific risk factors.*

Breast cells are exposed to a balance between the main sex hormones: estradiol, progesterone, testosterone, and *dihydrotestosterone.* Without this equilibrium, breast cancer frequently develops throughout a population. The grave consequences of the contraceptive pill have been known for more than thirty years [2]:

Consequences of Oral Contraceptive Use with A Decrease in Androgen Ovarian Synthesis	
Thrombosis of the deep veins [2]	Hypertension (140/90) * after five years of continuous use (5 percent of cases) [2]
Pulmonary embolism (risks × 2–12) [2]	Disturbances of the plasma lipoproteins [2]
Cerebral thromboembolism (risks × 3–9) [2]	Resistance to insulin [2]
Cerebral hemorrhage (risks ×2) [2]	
Breast cancer risk	[3] [4] [5] [6]
Sexual health complaints	[7]

Table 9

* The blood pressure has two digits which correspond to the maximum and minimum pressure. The upper digit may not exceed 120 mm of mercury. The lower digit may not exceed 80 mm of mercury. See hypertension page 140, table 1.

Breast Cancer Risk and Contraceptive Pill

A contraceptive pill is, in general, composed of estrogen along with a progestin. Sometimes progestin derivatives are used alone.

The use of the contraceptive pill breaks the balance of sex hormones.

In 2001, researchers at the Department of Oncology, Karolinska Hospital, Stockholm, Sweden, demonstrated in the following:

- Progestogens may be proliferative in breast tissue.
- Increased proliferation during hormonal contraception is an unwanted and potentially hazardous side effect.
- Women using oral contraceptives had significantly lower serum androgen levels compared with naturally cycling women—cell proliferation is more critical when testosterone levels are low.
- In certain women, after two months of oral contraceptive use, the percentage of proliferative cells was as high as 40 to 50 percent [3].

In 2006, Mayo Clinic Proceedings published a meta-analysis study by Kahlenborn and collaborators from the Department of Internal Medicine, Altoona Hospital, Altoona, Pennsylvania. This study concluded that the use of oral contraceptives is associated with an increased risk of premenopausal breast cancer, especially with use before the first full-term pregnancy in parous women [4].

In 2012, Li and his collaborators from the Division of Public Health Sciences, Fred Hutchinson Cancer Research Center, Seattle, Washington, published a study about the effect of depo-medroxyprogesterone acetate on breast cancer risk among women twenty to forty-four years of age in a large population [5]. This study confirmed the dangers of progesterone use in female contraception.

Depo-medroxyprogesterone acetate is an injectable contraceptive that contains a *progestin* that was found to increase breast cancer risk, when used as a menopausal hormone therapy regimen, among postmenopausal women in the Women's Health Initiative clinical trial conducted from 1993 to 1998 at forty clinical centers [6]. The 2012 study of Li and his collaborators found that injectable depo-medroxyprogesterone acetate use for twelve months or longer was associated with a 2.2-fold-increased risk of invasive breast cancer [5].

In conclusion, there is no doubt that the use of a contraceptive pill or the injectable contraceptive depo-medroxyprogesterone acetate breaks the balance of testosterone and dihydrotestosterone and leads to breast cancer.

Oral contraceptive use, however, has also been associated with women's sexual health complaints and androgen insufficiency. Oral contraceptive use is associated with a decrease in ovarian androgen synthesis and an increase in the production of sex hormone-binding globulin (SHBG) even months after stopping its use. Troubles may persist after stopping oral contraception [7].

What about a new contraceptive pill that uses a combination of estetrol and drospirenone?

Major pharmaceutical companies are now afraid to sell estrogen in combination with progestins because they have paid billions of dollars for damages caused by this pharmaceutical formula, which can cause breast cancer. They are right to be afraid.

With the resignation of the major pharmaceutical companies, some pharmacists are trying to get around the problem by doing the same thing by combining estetrol with drospirenone.

What Is Drospirenone?

Drospirenone is a progestin—a synthetic progestogen—and hence it acts like progesterone. It has antiandrogenic activity and no other important hormonal activity.

What Is Estetrol?

Estetrol (E4) is an estrogenic steroid molecule discovered in 1965. It is a weak estrogen synthesized exclusively by the fetal liver during human pregnancy. It reaches the maternal circulation through the placenta [8]. Its effects are dose-dependent, and 10 mg of estetrol has the same results as 2 mg of estradiol valerate, according to a 2017 publication [9].

In rats, estetrol has a protective effect on chemical-induced breast tumors and was found to reduce the number and size of breast tumors in a dose-dependent manner over treatment for eight weeks.

From there, pharmacists have imagined utilizing estetrol in contraceptive pills to replace more proliferative estrogens like estradiol. It can be exciting to be a step closer to discovering a safe solution for female contraception that avoids the risk of breast cancer. The contraceptive pill containing estetrol needs to be associated with a progestogen. The mixing of estetrol with drospirenone constitutes a problem, however. Breast cancer risks are associated with the use of progesterone alone [5] and with progestogens in combination with estrogens [6].

In any case, the estetrol-drospirenone pill does not alleviate the side effects that can be produced by the *inhibition of the total production of testosterone and dihydrotestosterone,* as with any contraceptive pill.

Testosterone production by the ovaries is always, in general, more significant than estradiol production [10]. Properly speaking, testosterone is not a sex hormone; it is an anabolic hormone in men and women, responsible for constructing the body structures. Testosterone needs to be transformed into dihydrotestosterone—the real sex hormone in men and women. No dihydrotestosterone, no sex hormone. Testosterone is also the chemical precursor of estradiol. When testosterone is delivered to the body, a part of it is transformed into estradiol, the proliferative hormone.

It is entirely incomprehensible that the clinical studies on contraceptives focus on estrogens and progestogens without considering the essential production of testosterone by the ovaries in young women. The contraceptive pill suppresses the secretions of all ovarian steroids, including estrogens, progesterone, and testosterone, which provokes a decrease of dihydrotestosterone production and its consequences: depression, urination problems, and decreased libido.

A blood check of plasma hormone concentrations is easy to do. Plasma hormone concentrations (nanograms/100 mL) in a woman before menopause are as follows:

Testosterone	57 ± 19 ng/100 mL
Dihydrotestosterone	**27 ± 6 ng/100 mL**

Table 10

A woman who, per 100 mL, has 57 ng of testosterone + 27 ng of dihydrotestosterone = 84 ng of androgens does not show androgen deficiency (on average).

A woman who, per 100 mL, has 19 ng of testosterone + 6 ng of dihydrotestosterone = 25 ng of androgens has androgen deficiency, less than a third of the standard level (on average).

Therefore, in all cases, it is useful to measure at least testosterone and dihydrotestosterone in the blood. A more detailed biological study is sometimes necessary to consider or follow a hormonal treatment.

The production of dihydrotestosterone represents a significant proportion of the circulating androgens (see previous discussion and chapter 5). Targets in sex organs and pilosity make this hormone.

Twenty-five-year-old women do not usually have breast cancer. Their androgen production is at its maximum. Thus, androgen production could prevent breast cancer from developing, with the hormonal balance being intact.

The key message of the World Health Organization is that *early detection to improve breast cancer outcome and survival remains the cornerstone of breast cancer control.*

For prevention and control of breast cancer, I suggest checking testosterone and dihydrotestosterone levels in women over the age of twenty-five, every year. The diagnosis for a compensatory treatment with mesterolone is then a possibility. This will advantageously replace clinical and radiological examinations from the age of forty because the prevalence of breast cancer will probably have decreased considerably. As an example, scurvy is no longer a significant threat because we know that we must take vitamin C. Diagnostic efforts and treatment should be aimed at hormonal correction of the causes of breast cancer, which would be much more profitable than looking for existing tumors. Because all contraceptive pills cause a severe drop in ovarian testosterone production, provoking depression, urination problems, decreased libido, and even breast cancer, it seems logical to produce contraceptive pills that contain a physiological quantity of androgens. All combinations of estrogens with progesterone should combine five or ten milligrams of mesterolone.

Without testosterone, the fluidity of the blood decreases in many cases, causing thrombosis (the secretion of antithrombin and other fluidity factors may be reduced). Without testosterone and dihydrotestosterone, brain function can be depressed.

The Contraceptive Pill That Most Suppresses Androgen Production

The contraceptive pill that most suppresses androgen production contains cyproterone—a very potent antiandrogen. It is used to combat the excess of pilosity or acne in women presenting with polycystic ovary syndrome (PCOS), the most common endocrine pathology in women of childbearing age.

In short, the use of this pill destroys all structures in the body that depend on androgens. The risk of suffering from phlebitis and pulmonary embolism is four times higher in women using these pharmaceutical compositions compared with women using conventional oral contraceptives. Therefore, these pharmaceutical compositions are sometimes not allowed for individual patients.

If women are considering using a contraceptive pill, *they should not trust the brand literature alone.* If the pill contains cyproterone, they should ask several medical professionals for advice.

The Best Birth Control Pill

A contraceptive pill always inhibits the production of testosterone by the ovaries. The best birth control pill should incorporate testosterone to replace the missing testosterone, thus protecting dihydrotestosterone production. But this formulation has technical difficulties. This is why, for technical reasons, the best contraceptive pill will have to contain five or ten milligrams of mesterolone. This contraceptive pill does not yet exist and needs further investigation [16].

Premenopause and Contraception

In the case of premenopause and contraceptive use, the balance between estradiol and progesterone could be impaired, leading to fibromyoma of the uterus, spotting, and bleeding. Androgen deficiencies exist in those cases because the expected testosterone concentration in the blood of a woman of age forty would be about half that of a woman of age twenty-one [11]. Considering that point, it is not surprising that women around forty who are taking a contraceptive pill that has antiandrogen effects will have more troubles than a woman of twenty whose ovaries produce reasonable amounts of androgens.

Artificial Menopause—Continuous and Extended Contraception

Continuous hormonal contraception stops menstruation, producing artificial menopause. The word *menopause* signifies the cessation of menstruation.

Some gynecological diseases can benefit from continued hormonal contraception. In 2007, the Canadian Society of Gynaecologists and

Obstetricians published t the *Consensus Guideline on Continuous and Extended Hormonal Contraception*. The words *testosterone* and *dihydrotestosterone* are not mentioned once [12].

A meta-analysis was done in 2014, "The Effect of Combined Oral Contraception on Testosterone Levels in Healthy Women: A Systematic Review and Meta-Analysis," which concluded: "The clinical implications of suppressed androgen levels during COC [combined oral contraceptives] use remain to be elucidated" [13]. Continuous contraception may induce deficiencies in testosterone and dihydrotestosterone. The resulting syndrome is then comparable to androgenic menopausal disease (chapter 1).

Warning

The administration of all pharmaceutical compositions that combine estrogen with a progestogen to provide contraception will inevitably lead to similar conditions of tumors or disorders, which are indexed in the following table and will invariably lead to new legal proceedings in the future [14,15].

Prudence would suggest that all compositions of estrogen with a progestin should indicate in their instructions for use that these associations can cause the disorders listed in table 11 secondary to inhibition of the production of testosterone and dihydrotestosterone.

All kinds of estrogen compositions with a progestin should indicate in their instructions for use that a dosage of testosterone and dihydrotestosterone should be made during contraception if there are any of the disorders listed in the table 11.

Similarly, the directions for use should specify that the desired contraception cannot be achieved by estrogen with progestin compositions if there are preexisting symptoms that predict the

Possible Complications of Oral Contraception Using Estrogen Compositions with a Progestin That May Cause a Decrease in Androgenic Secretions (Testosterone and Dihydrotestosterone)
• Headaches • Mood swings or depressed mood • Weight gain • Abdominal or pelvic pain, stomach pain, nausea • Breast sensitivity • Urinary problems: chronic cystitis, incontinence, urgency • Deep vein thrombosis • Pulmonary embolism • Cerebral thrombosis or embolism • Hemorrhage • High blood pressure • Plasma lipoprotein disorders • Insulin resistance • Possibility of inducing breast cancer

Table 11

existence of testosterone or dihydrotestosterone deficiencies. Because testosterone is a *precursor of estradiol*, it cannot be used in combination with a progestin composition because it will increase estradiol production. Finally, it will be useful for the pharmaceutical industry to inform the consumer about the possibility of a contraceptive pill that could avoid disasters caused by the lack of testosterone and dihydrotestosterone secretions (table 11). It is a contraceptive pharmaceutical composition that mixes a *progestin with mesterolone* to compensate for the deficit in testosterone and dihydrotestosterone produced by the progestin or the estrogen-progestin combination. Mesterolone has properties of testosterone and dihydrotestosterone. To avoid disasters, an estrogen-progestin or a progestin contraceptive pill should include mesterolone *at physiological doses* (5–10 mg/day). The new birth control pill does not yet exist. However, it will be easy to conduct studies leading to the pill's development [16].

This new model of pharmaceutical composition may very well constitute the treatment of PCOS associated with excess androgen production, which affects 10 percent of women. The estrogen-progestin–mesterolone contraceptive would suppress excessive androgen production (which results in acne and hirsutism) and replace it with physiological doses of androgens, thanks to the properties of mesterolone. To date, no treatment can cure PCOS.

All kinds of estrogens, alone or in combination with progestogens, may produce a premature androgenic disease.

Premature menopause or early menopause also causes premature genital aging (chapter 31).

Part III

Diseases of Aging

Androgenic disease of menopause
is a systemic disease
affecting all structures of the body
through various mechanisms

Testosterone is a systemic hormone.

Testosterone works on the metabolism of all nutrients:

- Sugars
- Fats
- Proteins

Testosterone is necessary for the right condition and proper functioning of the following:

- Heart
- Arteries and veins
- Joint articulations
- Brain
- Bladder and kidneys
- Immune system
- Masculine genitalia
- Skin

Androgenic disease of menopause is a systemic disease responsible for many diseases of aging.

8

Diabetes and Androgenic Menopausal Disease: The Sugar Mechanism

Key Facts

The World Health Organization (WHO) notes the following diabetes facts:

- The number of people with diabetes rose from 108 million in 1980 to 422 million in 2014.
- The global prevalence of diabetes among adults over eighteen years of age rose from 4.7 percent in 1980 to 8.5 percent in 2014.
- Diabetes prevalence has been growing more rapidly in the middle- and low-income countries.
- Diabetes is a significant cause of blindness, kidney failure, heart attacks, stroke, and lower limb amputation.
- In 2016, an estimated 1.6 million deaths were directly caused by diabetes. Another 2.2 million deaths were attributable to high blood glucose in 2012.
- Almost half of all deaths due to high blood glucose occur before the age of seventy years; the WHO estimates that diabetes was the seventh-leading cause of death in 2016.
- A healthy diet, regular physical activity, maintaining average body weight, and avoiding tobacco use are ways to prevent or delay the onset of type 2 diabetes.

- Diabetes can be treated, and its consequences can be avoided or delayed with diet, physical activity, medication, and regular screening and treatment for complications.

The WHO predicts that in 2030, diabetes will be the seventh-leading cause of death in the world [1].

Diabetes in Women and Testosterone

Few longitudinal studies of testosterone in women exist [2]. The reason is that women are associated with the female hormones; however, each day, a woman secretes more male hormones than female hormones, and this fact is not taught to or acknowledged by most doctors. Consequently, there are scarce available data about testosterone in women. Notwithstanding recently published contradictory studies, the existing studies are few.

Effects of Testosterone on Blood Sugar Levels Are the Same in Men and Women

In 1947, Giuseppe Pellegrini [3] proved that the administration of male hormones decreased the level of blood sugar in individuals with diabetes in an article entitled "The Antidiabetic Action of Male Sex Hormones within the Framework of Diabetes' Physiology" (published in Italian). The clinical study involved sixty-eight patients, some of whom were women. The intramuscular injection of testosterone was found to reduce the level of blood sugar in individuals with diabetes. This reduction occurred gradually, over two or three hours, following the administration of male hormones and acted until the fourth or fifth hour. The rates of glycosuria decreased simultaneously. The reduction of blood sugar was higher than one gram per liter of plasma.

In 2001, the National Institute of Health and Medical Research (INSERM) in France showed the improvement of the sensitivity to insulin with the administration of androgens [4]. This fascinating study demonstrated the efficacy of androgens in men to correct blood sugar in people with diabetes, emphasizing the importance of dihydrotestosterone. It would be useful, now and without delay, to do similar studies in women using mesterolone.

The Sugar Mechanism

The human body needs energy to function. The food contains three great sources of energy—sugars, fats, and proteins. The power (fuel) that is supplied immediately exists in sugars and fats. Glucose (sugar) is used instantaneously by the organism's cells. Proteins play a specific role, as we will see later.

Billions of glucose molecules cross the organism's cells at every moment. They are an energy source that is immediately usable by each cell. Parts of sugars are stored in the liver and muscles to constitute a reserve for use during strenuous efforts or periods of fasting. The assimilation of sugars is done immediately or slowly, according to their compositions. "Fast" sugars (e.g., the sugar in honey and extremely concentrated granulated sugar) are quickly digested by the intestines, causing an immediate rise in blood sugar levels, and are used immediately by the organism. "Slow" sugars (e.g., the starch in bread, pasta, and potatoes) are composed of subunits of glucose that are released gradually during digestion in the intestine. They raise blood sugar levels slowly for a longer period.

Fat contains fatty acids; fats include butter, margarine, and oils, such as sunflower oil, groundnut oil, and olive oil.

Fatty acids give fats their essential characteristics. They are soluble in fat solvents (e.g., acetone, ether, benzene) and are insoluble in water. Everyone knows that it is impossible to make grease stains on clothes disappear by washing them with water. They should be degreased by dry cleaning, which uses petrol or other grease solvents.

Glycerol (glycerin) is present in abundance in fats. It is a colorless liquid with a syrupy, sweetened taste and is soluble in alcohol.

Lipids constitute the essence of cell membranes. They play a significant role in the exchange of the molecules coming from the external world and their transport within the cell. In the brain, fats constitute the electrical insulation of nerves.

Fats are an essential energy source. All cells can store them, but they are mainly stored by fat cells.

An adult weighing 155 pounds has an energy reserve of 33 pounds of fat, 13 pounds of proteins, and 300 grams of carbohydrates (sugars). Seventy-two percent of the remaining weight consists of water. Fatty tissue represents the principal energy reserve of the organism (90 percent).

As noted, food sugar acts immediately. In excess, it penetrates fat cells, which transform it into fat. The fat in food is conveyed directly to fatty tissue, contributing to the accumulation of reserves. If the sugary food supply is missing, the organism automatically takes from its fat reserves to provide the necessary energy. This mobilization releases glycerol, which transforms into glucose, without which life is not possible. Indeed, whereas other parts of the body can use various energy sources, the brain permanently consumes *only glucose* (100–150 grams per day). A lack of glucose, as with a lack of oxygen, destroys the brain in a few minutes.

The level of sugar in the blood is constant. It results from a balance between the food supplies of sugar, the synthesis of glycogen by the liver, and its use by the muscles.

This balance is only possible as a result of regulation by various hormones. The traditional conceptualization recognizes hormones that raise the blood sugar and others that lower the blood sugar.

Blood sugar levels must imperatively remain constant with an empty stomach. The rise in blood sugar levels caused by food is immediately regularized by insulin, which brings the blood sugar back to the average level of below 140 milligrams per hundred cubic centimeters of plasma. However, insulin secretion can be insufficient, causing poor combustion of sugar, and the sugar level in the blood will remain high. A simple test makes it possible to confirm an insufficiency of insulin secretion. After ingesting seventy-five grams of glucose, the blood sugar must remain lower than or equal to two hundred milligrams per hundred cubic centimeters of plasma (two measurements are necessary). If one of the two measures is higher than two hundred milligrams of glucose per hundred cubic centimeters of plasma, the diagnosis of intolerance to glucose is a possibility. This diagnosis can reveal a predisposition to a severe disease: diabetes.

When the level of blood sugar exceeds 180 per hundred cubic centimeters of plasma, molecules of glucose cross the renal filter and are eliminated in the urine.

Ancient writings from Sushruta (six hundred years before Jesus Christ) contain what is probably the first description of diabetes: “When the doctor affirms that the man emits urine comparable with honey, he is declared incurable.” In the seventeenth and eighteenth centuries, tasters of urine existed; these individuals highlighted the presence of sugar in the urine.

In 1923, Banting and Best discovered insulin, which allows the hormonal control of sugar's metabolism, causing remarkable progress in the treatment of diabetic diseases.

A defect in insulin secretion can strike young women under thirty years of age. Such women suffer from a rare type of abnormal assimilation of sugars, insulin-dependent diabetes, which is determined by hereditary factors.

The vast majority of diabetes cases develop after forty years of age (more than 75 percent), and the frequency of diabetes in the Western population varies between 5 and 25 percent. Many factors contribute to the appearance of diabetes, but the cause is poorly defined. Dietary modification is essential to prevent and treat this severe affliction.

Diabetes causes multiple complications: pruritus (often localized at the genitals), repeated infections, eye troubles (e.g., cataracts), cardiac disorders (e.g., angina pectoris), vascular diseases (e.g., hypertension and gangrene), and nervous disorders (e.g., neuralgias and polyneuritis).

In the United States, diabetes is the third-leading cause of mortality and the number-one cause of blindness. In individuals with diabetes, the coronary risk is multiplied by four. An individual with diabetes who is older than age forty is obese in 80 percent of cases. Premature death from diabetes is directly connected to economic development in various areas of the world. In most countries, diabetes ranks between fourth and eighth in causes of mortality.

Classic theories acknowledge a necessary balance between hormones to maintain the constancy of blood sugar levels. Can one ask why the need for *testosterone* is unknown? Testosterone takes part in the determination of blood sugar levels because it allows the penetration of glucose into the muscles and the liver, thus decreasing blood sugar levels. Conversely, a lack of male hormones produces a rise in blood sugar levels.

A permanent lack of testosterone in a woman with androgenic menopausal disease causes a rise in blood sugar at every moment. This upsets the sugar balance, with an immediate consequence: insulin release to bring the blood sugar levels back to normal, provoking a feeling of hunger, commonly called a "need for sugar." The woman eats the first food she finds as a preferable source of fast sugars, to calm the feeling of hunger quickly. Again, this provokes a reaction of insulin, producing a vicious circle that will have no end. These phenomena explain, in women with androgenic menopausal disease, the symptoms of excess weight, obesity, and a tendency toward diabetes. Without an iron will, it is practically impossible to diet for prolonged periods. With the incapacity of doctors to solve the problem, we see the commercial exploitation of weight excess and obesity by charlatans, such as the diffusion of fad diets, which are all claimed to be more effective than the others, or by books that are little more than cookbooks.

Insulin acts with remarkable speed. An excess can cause death as a result of the sharp drop in blood glucose because the brain has a permanent need for glucose. The action of insulin does not last more than twenty-four hours, at which point the blood sugar levels go back to the initial values, and new insulin injections are necessary.

Male hormones act more slowly on the level of blood glucose. When prolonged treatment stops in a person with diabetes, the basal blood sugar (with an empty stomach) returns to the pathological values that preceded the treatment with male hormones.

Why Do Women Gain Weight after Age Forty?

Androgenic disease of menopause (in addition to overeating) is responsible for the vast majority of fatty diabetes and sugar intolerance after age forty. It causes an excess of weight and obesity for chemical reasons, worsened by ignorance about good diets.

As noted, the secretion of male hormones decreases after age twenty-five.

Each sugar release in the blood causes a strong reaction of insulin, which stores sugar in fats. The promptness of this reaction goes beyond what is necessary and makes the blood sugar level fall below average, resulting in hunger, discomfort, and the call for sugar. The vicious cycle is engaged and will develop with time.

No one can break this abnormal cycle without regulating male hormones. Therefore, a woman with androgenic disease of menopause is generally unable to control her weight, regardless of her efforts or goodwill. Always under the influence of discomfort, she finally abandons any rational alimentation, which is impossible to sustain over the long term.

A healthy diet, regular physical activity, the maintenance of a standard weight, and quitting smoking in association with the substitution of well-proportioned male hormones make it possible to prevent or delay the appearance of type 2 diabetes.

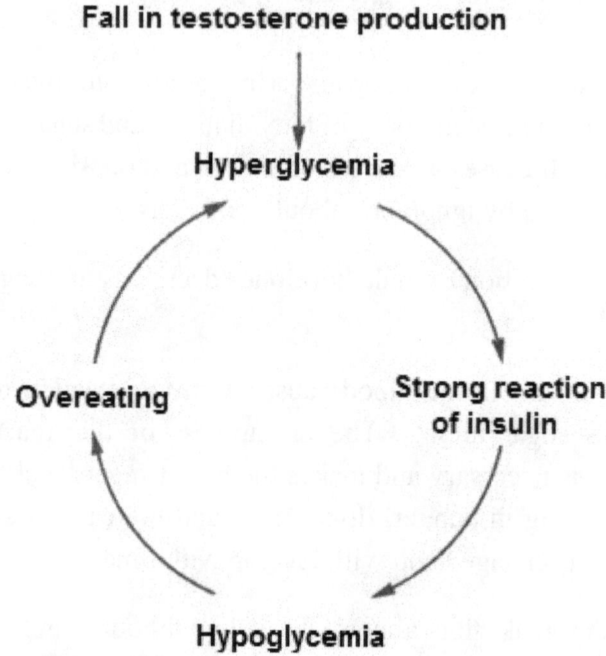

The abnormal cycle of glucose metabolism (simplified diagram).

As the secretion of male hormones continues to decrease over the years, the abnormal cycle of hyperglycemia, sugar, reaction and insulin release, hunger, and overeating accelerates, leading to excess weight, obesity, and ultimately, death.

9

Male Hormones against Cholesterol

Scientific studies on cholesterol are numerous and continuously evolving. This chapter simply draws attention to *one of the mechanisms* of increased cholesterol in the blood with age: the lack of male hormones that induces an elevation of glucose and, consequently, a rise in blood cholesterol in general.

Poor combustion of sugar and unbalanced food intake produce two well-known phenomena of age: accumulation of cholesterol and fats (triglycerides) in the blood. The measurement of cholesterol and blood triglycerides is part of the classic medical checkup. Everyone has heard about the cholesterol of one's grandfather or the triglycerides of one's grandmother. There is no day when the medical press does not evoke the need for controlling the rise of fats in the blood, which increases cardiovascular risk.

It is probably Poulletier de la Salle who isolated, in 1769, the first well-defined lipid, cholesterol, present in gallstones.

In the United States, sixteen to twenty million individuals have gallstones, made up of 80 percent cholesterol. Autopsies showed that at least 8 percent of men had gallstones and at least 20 percent of women. Each year, one million new cases appear.

Cholesterol comes partly from food, but the liver manufactures the most significant quantity. Its excess in the blood is the expression of a self-destruction mechanism inherent to the organism.

Fat is a source of energy. Cholesterol in excess is accumulated and stored by the body; its elimination is done almost exclusively by the liver, which excretes it in the bile, where it can crystallize in the form of gallstones.

The balance between the entry and exit of cholesterol is essential to maintain the constancy of the interior medium. If entries are more than needed, cholesterol accumulates in the arteries and fat deposits under the skin (xanthomas).

The formation of cholesterol comes primarily from the liver. Food is a secondary source of the contribution; the intestines absorb only 40 percent of food cholesterol. These characteristics explain why a diet, regardless of type, is unable to cause a significant drop in blood cholesterol because the intestines assimilate relatively little.

Cholesterol plays a central role in the human body. It takes part in the formation of the cellular membranes, for example.

It is starting from the cholesterol molecule that hormones (steroids) are manufactured by the suprarenal glands and by the testicles. The action of testosterone, the hormone of construction, is permanently against cortisol, which opposes its action. Testosterone increases the synthesis of proteins, from the Greek *protos*, which means "first," which are essential substances for the organism. They have exceptional biological properties.

Cortisol coming from the suprarenal glands decreases the synthesis of proteins. Testosterone reduces the blood sugar level; cortisol increases it. It is enough to understand that these two hormones act in opposite directions.

Cholesterol is an alcohol that is in a free state in the cells of the organism, where it makes hormones or components of cellular membranes. It also has the property of retaining water in the cells and preventing them from desiccation. Manufactured by the liver, it is moved toward the cells of the organism.

In the plasma, 80 percent of cholesterol is related to fatty acids. It is the *"bad" cholesterol* that deposits in the form of fats in the arterial walls when it is in excess in the blood.

Fats are insoluble in water. To be transported in the blood, which is aqueous, they bind to proteins (lipoproteins), whose properties enable them to circulate.

Low-density lipoprotein (LDL), a specific lipoprotein, transports the *bad cholesterol.*

"Good" cholesterol is not bound to fatty acids; it is not fat. It comes from the combustion of the unhealthy cholesterol, released of its fatty acids, and represents 27 percent of the total cholesterol in a man aged twenty to twenty-four. A specific lipoprotein does its transport, high-density lipoprotein (HDL), charged with collecting cholesterol in sites where it is in excess and transporting it toward the liver, where it is degraded and excreted in the form of biliary acid.

The rise in blood cholesterol levels also depends on a whole series of factors that are not within the framework of this book.

An increase in blood cholesterol with age, in the same population with the same dietary habits, poses the problem of an essential cause accentuated with time.

The lipid research program of the National Institutes of Health in the United States defines the average cholesterol level in the population. These results were derived from values determined in eleven communities [1].

Table 12 shows that the rise in blood cholesterol primarily starts with bad cholesterol (LDL cholesterol). It is the bad cholesterol that increases with age. There is a storage of toxic fats. The cause of this accumulation of bad cholesterol is the abnormal cycle of sugar combustion, started by the insufficiency of male hormones secretion in the woman after age twenty-five.

Average Values of Blood Cholesterol According to Age in the United States			
Age	Total Plasma Cholesterol in mg/100 mL	Plasma LDL Cholesterol in mg/100 mL	Plasma HDL Cholesterol in mg/100 mL
20–24	162	103	45
25–29	179	117	45
30–34	193	126	46
35–39	201	133	43
40–44	205	136	44
45–49	213	144	45
50–54	213	142	44

Table 12

From the US National Institutes of Health [1].

A lack of male hormones causes sugar excess, which automatically generates the synthesis of bad cholesterol because the organism's capacities for the elimination of cholesterol are limited.

Accumulation of bad cholesterol by the body is the result of two different but complementary phenomena. The first is overeating, which increases the glucose contribution. The second is the continued manufacturing of cholesterol, starting from an excess of glucose. Bad cholesterol, not eliminated sufficiently, deposits in the arterial walls.

Triglycerides (Fats)

Triglycerides are reserve substances stored by specialized cells, the adipocytes. They are found under the skin, around the abdominal organs in a kind of fatty apron (epiploon) covering the intestines, and in many areas of the organism.

These fats are used as heat insulators (obese individuals suffer less from cold than do thin people) and protect the body against shocks. Triglycerides are a reserve of energy. These reserves are fuel for the organism. They are transported remotely to be "burned" where they are necessary (thanks to very-low-density lipoprotein [VLDL], which also conveys a small portion of bad cholesterol).

Triglyceride levels practically double between twenty and fifty years of age in the fat mass of humans. In a study relating to a population having mostly the same food lifestyle, one can suspect the existence of a fundamental cause that accentuates its harmful effects with age.

The accumulation of triglycerides (fats) is a process similar to that which determines the accumulation of cholesterol. It acts twice: initially, the collection of glucose by the abnormal cycle *and then the transformation of glucose into triglycerides* via *the acetyl-coenzyme A.*[*] Triglycerides accumulate in fat tissue for a long time as the food supplies remain excessive.

---

[*] Glucose is "burned" (energy production) by the organism in a series of chemical reactions, called the Krebs cycle, that produces a molecule, acetyl-coenzyme A, from which cholesterol is formed.

Many scientific works showed the favorable influence of male hormones on the regulation of cholesterol and triglycerides. Good cholesterol (HDL) is higher in the blood of men having raised levels of male hormones [2,3].

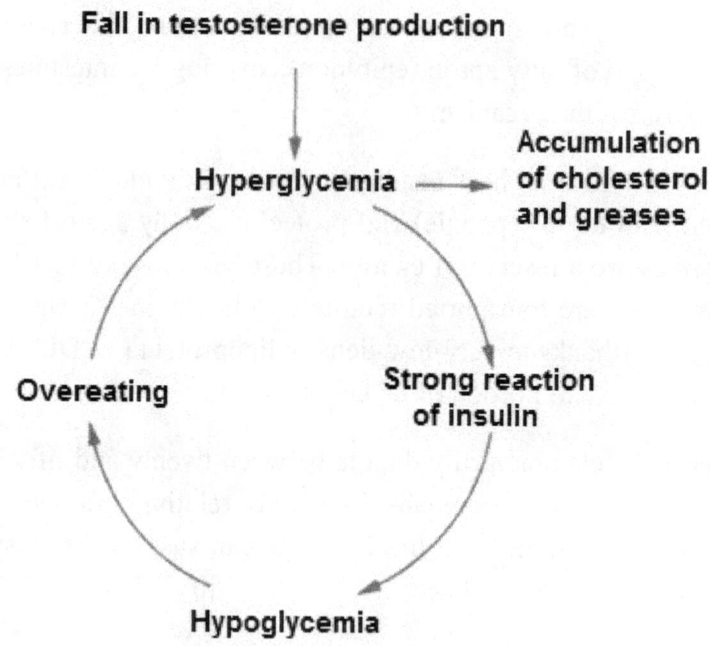

Accumulation of cholesterol and fats in a woman with androgenic menopausal disease (simplified diagram).

The level of blood triglycerides depends on the mobilization of fat reserves and the food supply. The National Institutes of Health in the United States determined the average triglyceride levels in the blood according to age [1], as shown in table 13.

A lack of male hormones causes sugar intolerance and diabetes and dangerously raised levels of cholesterol and fats, thus creating an increase in fat mass and obesity, all of which support the appearance of cardiovascular disease, the leading cause of mortality in the world.

Average Triglyceride Levels in Plasma According to Age	
Age	Triglycerides in mg/100 mL
20–24	89
25–29	104
30–34	122
35–39	141
40–44	152
45–49	143
50–54	154

Table 13

Blood triglyceride levels rise with age [1].

Atheroma

Atheroma is sometimes also called *atherosclerosis*. However, the latter term introduces some confusion with *arteriosclerosis*, which is an entire pathology (chapter 12). One should not confuse atherosclerosis (atheroma) and arteriosclerosis. *Atheroma* is an entirely suitable term.

In 1904, Marchand coined the word *atherosclerosis*—*atheroma* means “mash” in Greek—to indicate the fatty and fibrous degeneration of arteries. Eminent authorities contested this term.

Today, doctors regard atherosclerosis as an entity. *Atheroma* names the "atheromatous" form of arteriosclerosis—a pathology in which the mechanism is different from that which causes arteriosclerosis.

Localizations of Atheroma

Atheroma develops in places according to the localization of the deposits of fats, which appear in the form of fatty streaks, fibrous plates, or complicated lesions.

Fatty scratches appear, initially characterized by the accumulation of fats, mainly the cholesterol oleate, in the smooth muscle cells, and by the development of fibrous tissue under the internal tunic of the artery. These deposits are visible with the naked eye and can appear at any place in the arterial network. In all children, fatty traces are present in the aorta from ten years of age. At twenty-five years of age, they sometimes occupy 30 to 50 percent of the surface of the aorta. At this stage, the greasy deposits could reabsorb, but nothing makes it possible to affirm this.

The fibrous plates appear between thirty and forty years of age, and their number increases gradually with age. They develop primarily in the aorta, heart arteries, carotid arteries, and arteries flooding the brain. They consist of a core of fats, principally linoleate cholesterol, and the waste of dead cells, surrounded by many smooth muscle cells and collagen. The whole protrudes into the artery and causes turbulent zones in the bloodstream.

The complicated lesion is a plate encrusted with calcium, containing waste tissue and forming ulcers. While developing, it can completely obliterate the artery (stricture) and be the source of an embolism, starting from fragments that are detached and carried by the bloodstream. Lastly, the weakened and thinned arterial wall can break and cause internal bleeding.

The increase of fibrous plates and their complications with age poses the problem of a cause that worsens with time.

The Mechanism of Atheroma

The abnormal cycle of glucose excess causes overproduction of triglycerides and cholesterol in the blood (see chapters 8 and 9). Cholesterol in excess cannot leave the organism. Accompanied by fats, it diffuses in the internal walls of the arteries, preferring zones with blood turbulence, for example, the crossroads of the aorta. Consequently, it contacts the fibers of elastin. This protein, by its structure, has a strong affinity for fats and calcium. The elastic structures load cholesterol, fats, and calcium, losing their elasticity. The evolution of this process leads to the formation of atheroma.

When there is an atheroma, it is already too late, but one can improve on what remains useful in the arteries. It is necessary to prevent the formation of the atheroma at the beginning of the disease, avoiding the accumulation of bad cholesterol and fats. We saw the crucial role of male hormones and the need for rigorous food control in this regulation. One does not go without the other.

Control of one's nutrition is fundamental. Foods too rich in sugars and fats, and a lack of exercise, can cause the creation of atheromas.

Individual variations in the production of male hormones clarify sexual differences between individuals. They also explain why some individuals develop atheroma earlier than others.

In 1997, Hoffman and his collaborators showed that atherosclerosis is significantly associated with vascular dementia and Alzheimer's disease (see chapter 27) by measuring the relationship between the blood pressures in the arms and the ankles in a group of 284 people with dementia; the thickness of the carotid artery walls was determined by ultrasound [4].

10

Excess Weight and Obesity: The Ideal Weight

Impaired sugar and cholesterol mechanisms and overeating lead to overweight and obesity. Being overweight, caused by the accumulation of fats, starts, obviously, with the first extra kilo. In the beginning, this phenomenon is hardly perceptible. With time, the silhouette changes, kilo after kilo.

The excess weight gradually gives way to obesity when the overload reaches 20 percent of the body mass. The obesity of women is characteristic. Fat settles initially in the buttocks, then in the belly, and then invades the top of the body gradually.

The trunk and the shoulders thicken, and then the neck, the nape, and the face. The round and fatty face lose its expressivity because of the fat-covered mimic muscles. Fat deposits in the side parts of the eyelids are characteristic, giving a false air of sleepiness.

Obesity is a symptom, like a fever. There are major disordered states of metabolism that explain certain rare cases of obesity (the excessively large ones). In the vast majority of cases, however, the cause of being overweight is unknown. This explains the multiple therapeutic attempts, sometimes discouraging, that opened the field to charlatans. The phenomenon takes on worrying proportions in the United States and constitutes a real public health problem in the entire world. In terms of the frequency of obesity, the numbers speak for themselves. According to the World Health Organization (WHO), on a worldwide scale, the number of cases of obesity has doubled since 1980.

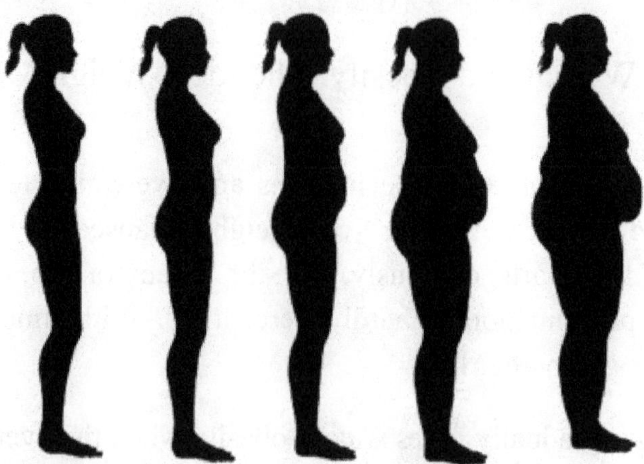

Fig. 18
Outline of a regressive woman: age twenty, twenty-five, thirty, forty, and fifty-five years.

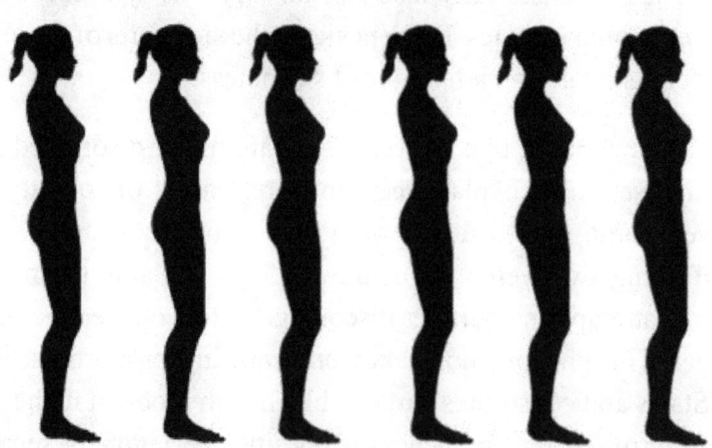

Fig.19

Outline of an ageless woman: twenty to eighty years.

In 2014, there were 1.9 billion overweight individuals eighteen years old or older. Of this total, six hundred million were obese (11 percent of men and 15 percent of women). Obesity affects nearly 41 million children of less than five years of age. According to the WHO, obesity is avoidable.

In the United States, 30 to 40 percent of the population is more than 10 percent overweight. This percentage progresses year by year and constitutes a challenge for the US government, which has engaged vast research programs to stop the catastrophe. Obesity is responsible for 1 to 3 percent of the total expenses for health in most countries (5 to 10 percent in the United States), and the costs will quickly increase in the years to come because obesity increases with diseases of aging.

Life insurance companies outline clear guidelines on obesity. The Metropolitan Life Insurance Company, for example, published weight tables fixing obesity at an increased body mass of 20 percent compared to an average person of the same sex and size.

Because the mortality of an obese woman is more likely than that of a woman having an ideal weight, she pays increased premiums on life insurance. The comparatively high death rate of those who are obese is worrying. Severely obese women die eight to ten years earlier than those with a standard weight, just like smokers. Thirty-three pounds of additional weight increases the risk of premature death by approximately 30 percent.

What Are the Classifications of Overweight and Obese?

Being overweight or obese is defined as an abnormal or excessive accumulation of body fat, which can harm health.

How does one determine an excess of weight? There are several formulas to calculate whether one is overweight by taking size into account. None is perfect because there are constitutional differences between individuals (e.g., a woman with strong bones and musculature is more massive). One of the most recent is the body mass index (BMI). This index divides the weight in kilograms by the height squared, expressed in meters.

BMI =	$\frac{\text{Weight (kilos)}}{\text{Height}^2 \text{ (meters)}}$

The WHO defines overweight and obesity as follows:

- Overweight is a BMI equal to or higher than twenty-five.
- Obese is a BMI equal to or higher than thirty.

In 1959, the ideal weight tables of the Metropolitan Life Insurance Company corresponded to a BMI of twenty-two; above twenty-two would be considered overweight.

It is necessary to get suitable treatment so as not to exceed this index level. Correction of weight is more accessible at the beginning of fat accumulation. It has even been said that an average excess of two pounds shortens one's life by two months.

What Is Your Ideal Weight?

One should consider the BMI formula to answer this question. The formula is as follows:

$$22 \times \text{height (in meters)}^2 = \text{ideal weight}$$

For example, for a height of 1.80 meters: $22 \times 1.82^2 = 22 \times 3.24 =$ 71.28 kilos (157.14 pounds) = ideal weight.

Thinness is also not a good sign. Lew and Garfinkel [1] showed, in a study relating to a population of 750,000 men and women, a higher death rate of individuals whose weight was lower than 10 percent of the standard weight.

Remaining thin as a result of a suitable diet, however, does not have the same meaning. Some even recommend systematic malnutrition to increase longevity. This approach could be under consideration, with the condition of not misusing the low-calorie diet that leads to thinness.*

Energy reserves are necessary to fight disease and to support a period of fasting. Whatever the diet, it must be balanced to maintain the right weight because obesity causes devastation.

Complications, whose frequency is well known, reduce the longevity of the obese.

---

* Thinness is the result of the disappearance, reduction, or insufficiency of the fat reserves of the organism, sometimes accompanied by atrophy of the muscular mass.

What Are the Most Frequent Consequences of Being Overweight or Obese?

A high BMI is a significant risk factor for chronic diseases, such as the following:

• Cardiovascular disease (mainly heart disease and stroke), which is the leading cause of death worldwide

• Diabetes

• Muscular and skeletal disorders (e.g., osteoarthritis, a degenerative disease of the joint articulations)

• Certain cancers (e.g., of the endometrium, breast, and colon)

Fat mass doubles between eighteen and fifty years of age and continues to increase. At the same time, muscular mass decreases. Simple observation makes it possible to note this. We know that testosterone secretion decreases after age twenty-five. This hormone is necessary for the maintenance of muscularity and fat mass. Bringing these phenomena together clarifies the cause and its consequences (other factors worsen the situation).

A progressive lack of male hormones can cause one to become overweight, which increases with age. All therapeutic efforts generally relate to the diet, particular food, and general measures. Nevertheless, the frequency of obesity continues to progress everywhere in the world. In individuals, it develops with time (figure 18).

Admittedly, through willpower, certain women manage to maintain their weight within reasonable limits thanks to a balanced diet and exercise. But all women do not have an iron will. Discouragement and relapses are the rule despite the desire to lose weight.

Old, frustrated obese women often deploy ingenuity and diet-program calculations, generally without result. Why this frustration? Women of less than age twenty usually eat anything and do not gain weight (figure 19). They have a maximum secretion of male hormones.

Male hormones cause the mobilization of reserve fats (lipolysis). The mechanism is complex and is beyond the scope of this text.

Clinical studies showed a decrease in male hormones in the obese. In 1990, Zumoff and his collaborators confirmed a reduction in the plasma free testosterone and total testosterone levels in the obese. The drop in the plasma level was proportional to the degree of obesity [2].

The human organism is perpetually in a situation of balance between construction and destruction. The treatment of obesity is, overall, a failure. The regulation of hormones is vital to ensure the stability of the body. However, chemistry cannot do everything. The following fact is of great importance: we are not obligated to eat four times a day (or more!). In the endeavor to manage weight, it is necessary to ensure calm for the brain.

It is illogical to think that food restriction only can suffice to ensure longevity. It is essential to reinforce the construction of the out-of-date fatty organism, which breaks up thanks to the hormone of life, testosterone, which is also the hormone of structure.

11

Muscular Weakness

Muscle contracts as a result of the energy brought by a sugar, glycogen, a muscle fuel. It is a complex molecule used as an energy reserve. Subunits of glucose make glycogen, an essential source of energy for the body. One finds it in honey, grapes, and fruits.

Blood sugar levels depend on the quantity of ingested sugar but also its release from muscle and liver reserves—even fat tissue stores glucose in the form of fatty acids and triglycerides.

In a healthy state, there is a balance between the blood levels of glucose and the reserves accumulated in the muscles and fat.

With an empty stomach, the average level of blood sugar is lower than 140 milligrams per hundred cubic centimeters of venous blood (two measurements are necessary to confirm constancy of the disordered state beyond 140) [1], with the ideal being around one hundred.

If one translates these milligrams into molecules,* that represents a billion molecules in circulation. Blood makes a complete turn through the organism in one minute; blood flow in organs is thus extremely high.

The healthy kidney comprises one hundred billion cells. One liter or two hundred cubic centimeters of blood irrigates this organ in one minute. So, in each minute, several billion molecules of glucose penetrate each cell [2].

---

* The molecule is the smallest particle of matter that preserves its characteristics.

This phenomenon is similar in the muscles, which permanently receive considerable quantities of glucose molecules, transformed and stored in the form of glycogen. Without it, muscle does not function, just as a car cannot run without gasoline. Glycogen is a muscle's fuel. It is permanently "burned" at the time of the muscular contraction.

The action of male hormones on muscular tissue has been known for many years. Male hormones penetrate the muscular cell, where they bind to a specific receptor, whose existence was shown by Jung and Beaulieu [3] and other authors. The hormone moves toward the cell nucleus, where it starts its hormonal effect. The essential reactions are of two types. Initially, the synthesis of proteins increases through the incorporation of new amino acids (the subunits of proteins). Then glycogen contents also increase significantly [4]. Hypertrophy of the muscle follows, as is well known by athletes who wish to improve their performance.

In an athlete, prolonged efforts increase the consumption of male hormones. Excessive use of male hormones during protracted physical efforts causes a lowering of the blood levels of male hormones, resulting in two principal consequences.

The first is psychological. The drop in the testosterone level in the blood causes a feeling of tiredness and depression, increasing with effort, leading finally to abandonment. The second is metabolic. The drop in blood testosterone prevents the recovery of energy stocks in the muscle. The fuel (glycogen) is missing—avoiding any extra effort, the athlete crumbles, unable to move.

In 2013, researchers in the Department of Endocrinology, Diabetes, and Nutrition of the Boston Medical Center showed the regeneration of skeletal muscle by testosterone in castrated mice [5]. Cellular regeneration and the proliferation of the cells were manifest four days after castration in young, two-month-old mice as in old, twenty-four-month-old mice.

An excess of male hormones increases the muscular mass beyond what is reasonable. The opposite is also exact: a lack of male hormones causes a reduction in the muscular mass and its atrophy.* Muscles, agents of motility, are atrophied in women with *androgenic menopausal disease*. An increase in fat and a decrease in muscular mass transform the body, which becomes soft instead of being firm. This fact leads to a reduction in the density of an older adult. Body density varies from 1,040 at around twenty years to 1,016 at approximately fifty years.

The physiological importance of endogenous testosterone in older women is poorly understood. Testosterone conversion into dihydrotestosterone in women is notably absent in numerous scientific studies. Nevertheless, the scarce experimental results have emphasized the role of testosterone in muscles in women.

In 2011, researchers from the Division of Endocrinology of the University of Pennsylvania School of Medicine, Philadelphia, Pennsylvania, published a study noting higher serum free testosterone concentrations in older women. High levels of testosterone correspond to greater bone mineral density, lean body mass, and total fat mass [6].

In 2014, a study from the Center for Human Nutrition, Division of Geriatrics and Nutritional Science, Department of Internal Medicine, Washington University School of Medicine, St. Louis, Missouri,

---

* Atrophy is characterized by a reduction in the volume of a living structure caused by deficient nutrition, lack of use, a physiological process of regression, and disease.

demonstrated that testosterone and progesterone, but not estradiol, stimulate muscle protein synthesis in postmenopausal women [7].

If estradiol is not necessary to develop the muscles of older women, then what is the need for "classic" hormone replacement therapy (HRT)?

The weakened musculature of older women is the result of *androgenic menopausal disease.* It is an indication for androgen therapy with mesterolone.

12

Arteriosclerosis or Arterial Rigidity

Popularly, arteriosclerosis is known as *arterial rigidity*. The definition from *Webster's New World College Dictionary* is as follows: "arteriosclerosis, an abnormal thickening, and loss of elasticity of arteries' walls. *Origin of arteriosclerosis* (arterio- + sclerosis)." But dictionaries sometimes give another definition that confuses *arteriosclerosis* with *atherosclerosis*. Healthy arteries are flexible and elastic, but over time, the walls of arteries can harden, a condition commonly called *hardening of the arteries*, sometimes restricting blood flow to organs and tissues.

Warning

The term *arteriosclerosis* refers to a precise pathology, and *atherosclerosis* is a different concept.

The definition of the 2016 edition of the *American Heritage Dictionary of the English Language* is as follows:

> atherosclerosis, a form of arteriosclerosis characterized by the presence of lesions (called plaques) on the innermost layer of the walls of large and medium-sized arteries. The plates contain lipids, collagen, inflammatory cells, and other substances and can impede blood flow or rupture, leading to severe problems such as heart attack or stroke—caused by *atherosclerosis*.

The term *atherosclerosis* was invented one day by an enlightened mind that confounded two arterial pathologies, the first caused by sclerosis of arterial walls, and the second caused by deposits of greasy plates in the light of these. In the first case, it is a disease. In the latter case, it is a syndrome (chapter 9).

Arteriosclerosis is a disease of aging that has a specific cause, specific consequences, and a particular treatment. In the medical literature, the reasons for arteriosclerosis are unknown.

Pathological cuts of a sclerosed artery show disorganization of muscle fibers and their replacement by rigid fibrous tissue (the tissue of scars). Arterial resistance to blood-wave propagation increases and causes hypertension upstream of the functional obstacle. The internal wall of the artery, subjected to a permanent excess of pressure, thickens, reducing the arterial diameter.

Arteriosclerosis is the keystone of cardiovascular disease. It constitutes the first cause of mortality in Western countries and the United States [1].

Before age sixty-five, men die more frequently from the complications of arteriosclerosis than women; after this age, degeneration strikes women as much as men.

Arteriosclerosis is a common phenomenon after age forty. It is the leading cause of mortality after age sixty-five. The eighty-year-old man generally presents with signs of arteriosclerosis. The expression "you are as old as your arteries" finds its significance here.

Mechanism of Arteriosclerosis

It is important not to confuse the mechanism of arteriosclerosis with that of atheroma in the following question: Why do arteries harden with age?

For some authors, arteriosclerosis is a typical degenerative process that accompanies aging; it is not a disease. This degeneration does not depend on risk factors. Others call upon the importance of diet; fats in blood; and the role of cigarette smoking, psychic stress, and other factors that can interact with the pathogenesis of arteriosclerosis. These elements, however, do not seem to explain the origin of arterial hardening. Hypertension, age concerns, and constitutional factors have also been called upon to explain arteriosclerosis. For many people, the cause of arteriosclerosis remains a mystery.

One element must draw our attention. Observation of histological cuts of sclerosed arteries can reveal some things. The pathologist will observe, without difficulty, that the lesions of arterial walls show characteristics of scar tissue. In arteriosclerosis, the conjunctive tissue replaces the muscle fibers. But what is the cause?

Muscular arteries regulate the arterial flow [2]. They constitute a genuine engine necessary for the propulsion of the blood wave. It contains proteins and glycogen that are the available energetic factors. When dynamic contributions decrease, with time, muscle fibers are less contractile and finally become too weak. They end up dying, being replaced by fibrous tissue containing rigid collagen, unable to propagate the blood wave.

The comparison with the ureter, which is also a conduit whose motility depends on its musculature, seems evident to me. The ureter whose muscle fibers have been replaced by sclerosed tissue is unable to propel urine. In the same circumstances, the artery will not be able to move the blood.

After nine years of study in a university pathology laboratory, I showed, in 1971, a comparable phenomenon in the ureter's wall at the place where it enters the bladder (the terminal ureter) [3, 4]. At that time, I wondered why some children presented with ureters that were very dilated (megaureter) without apparent cause. Urine accumulated in the dilated ureter and crossed with difficulty in its final segment, not seemingly narrowed. The phenomenon was often allotted to hypothetical nervous disorders. This anomaly involved the destruction of the kidneys, invariably caused by hypertension in the ureter. I compared the healthy structure of the normal terminal ureter with the segments unable to propagate the wave of urine in a pathological study involving more than fifty thousand histological cuts. In all cases, the musculature of the final ureter was defective, or the seat of malformations, and was replaced, generally, by rigid fibrous tissue unable to propagate the urinary wave [3, 4].

When a segment of the ureter is sclerosed, that involves an overload upstream. The ureter dilates above the obstacle. Its muscle fibers, subjected to excessive work, hypertrophy initially. Then, with time, these fibers become atrophied and are replaced by the fibrous tissue of the dilated ureter [5].

The phenomenon is similar in arteries, whose muscle fibers constitute an engine necessary to the propulsion of the blood wave.

When an arterial segment becomes fibrous anywhere in the arterial network, that involves extra work for the arterial musculature upstream. It hypertrophies initially and then is atrophied mechanically. To add to that, the muscle fibers of the whole arterial musculature degenerate from a lack of energy factors.

The arterial muscular engine, like any engine, cannot function without the contribution of energy in the form of proteins and glycogen.

The conjunctive tissue located between arteries' muscle fibers also becomes rigid as a result of the lack of male hormones (chapter 17).

Mesterolone normalizes the structure of muscle fibers. Under these conditions, arterial stiffness will not occur with aging. There will be no hypertension. And if there is no hypertension, no antihypertensive treatment will be necessary [6].

Arteriosclerosis is consequently the result of the following:

1. Degeneration of the muscle fibers of the artery from a lack of male hormones, thus preventing the incorporation of energy factors like proteins and glycogen in the arterial musculature

2. A rigidity of conjunctive arterial tissue from a lack of male hormones

3. An excess of pressure on the walls of the artery upstream from a rigid fibrous segment anywhere in the arterial network, causing the mechanical hypertrophy of the arterial musculature and then its atrophy and its replacement by fibrous tissue, in addition to its biological degeneration (see points 1 and 2).

This is a perfect example of the vicious pathological cycles that imply several pathogeneses.

All women and men are finally affected by arteriosclerosis one day or another because the hormonal production decreases gradually with age

The energy material (proteins and glycogen) suddenly goes missing in the arterial muscular structures. They degenerate quickly, replaced by rigid fibrous tissue. Consequently, the tiny arteries located at the end of the arterial network do not regularly supply blood to organs, including the eyes, ears, and hippocampus in Alzheimer's disease (chapter 27).

Doctors are confronted daily with the devastations of cardiovascular disease. An aspect of prevention consists of supervising the cholesterol levels of their patients and prescribing cholesterol-lowering drugs. They could improve the health of their patients by also managing male hormones when necessary. A woman having "good" biological results with her cholesterol under cholesterol-lowering drugs will inevitably develop arteriosclerosis as a result of a lack of male hormones.

The male hormone is a general concept that does not explain "what to do" and "how to do it." For example, testosterone is known as an androgen, but it is an anabolic hormone that needs to be converted into another one to be androgenic.

In the *Merriam-Webster* definition, an androgenic hormone is a steroid hormone, such as testosterone, that controls the development and maintenance of masculine characteristics. In this definition, the term *control* has a general meaning. A better description would be as follows: "an androgenic hormone is a steroid hormone, such as testosterone that could influence the development and maintenance of masculine characteristics." However, this definition is also too general.

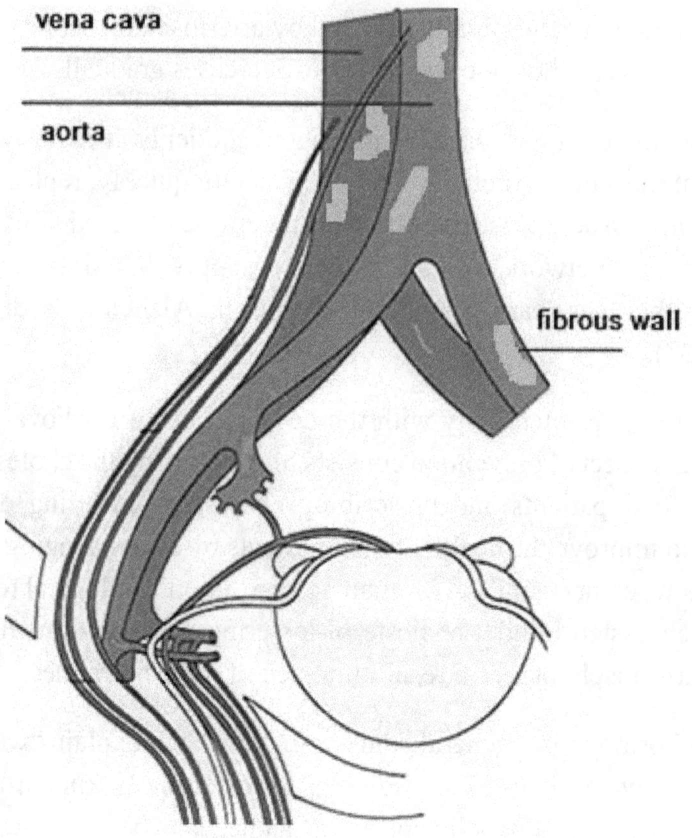

Fig. 21

The figure 21 shows areas at the beginning of their degeneration. Degenerating plaques of the aorta and iliac artery are shown in light grey. With age, the number of these fibrous areas will grow, and the fibrous tissue invades the entire arterial network. The muscle tissue of arteries degenerates.
A lack of muscle construction in men and women provokes the muscle degeneration.

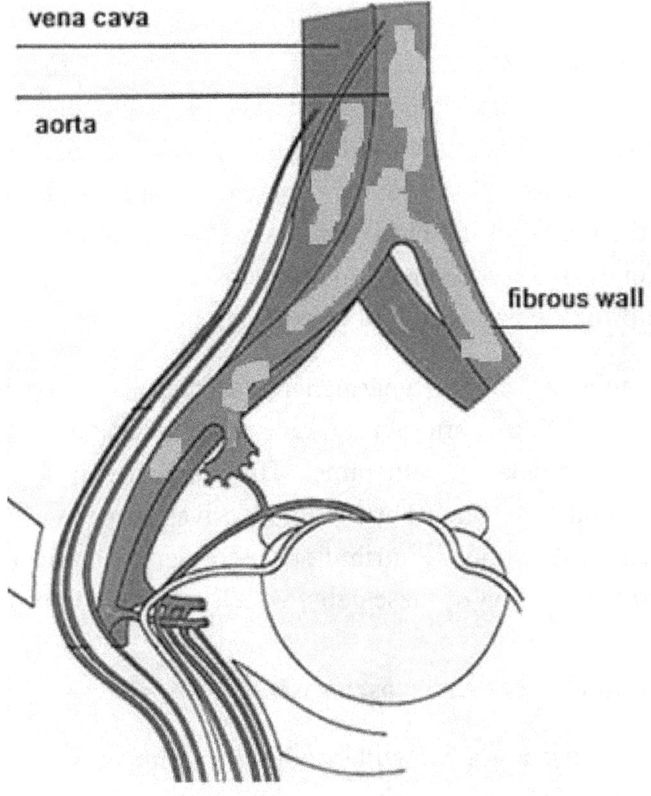

Fig. 22

Arteriosclerosis Is a Disease

- It has a cause, a lack of energetic factors for arterial muscle fibers.
- It has a direct consequence, the fibrosis of arterial muscle. (See fibrous tissue in light grey in the figure 22.
- It has a preventive daily permanent treatment for life with mesterolone from age forty and even before [6]

.

In a woman of age twenty, testosterone and dihydrotestosterone are well balanced. When there exists a lack of production with aging, for technical reasons, testosterone and dihydrotestosterone, which are then artificial hormones, may not be introduced in the body without provoking a biological disturbance; they are not approved for use in women by the US Food and Drug Administration (FDA), with reason. Thus, artificial testosterone and dihydrotestosterone are inappropriate and not valid for the prevention of arteriosclerosis.

Diseases of aging develop in a permanent vascular disorder caused by arteriosclerosis. The tiny arteries that constitute the end of the arterial network are particularly vulnerable. They are the first to have diminished blood flow. Their obstruction deprives the cells of oxygen, causing their destruction. Contributions of essential molecules are necessary to the survival of these cells, which are also compromised.

What to Do to Prevent Arteriosclerosis?

The preceding discussion notwithstanding, a solution does exist to prevent arteriosclerosis and its numerous complications, which include the following:

- Arterial hypertension
- Hearing and vision troubles (e.g., cataracts, retinal detachment, age-related macular degeneration)
- Angina pectoris
- Myocardial infarct
- Arterial rupture
- Vascular degeneration of joint articulations
- Renal insufficiency
- Arterial occlusion of lower extremities
- Parkinson's disease

- Alzheimer's disease
- Stroke

A lack of dihydrotestosterone is the first step in the deficiency of anabolic hormones. With mesterolone, a safe molecule, it possible to substitute the anabolic deficit around age forty or even before [6].

Indeed, dihydrotestosterone is a final hormone of androgen production. Testosterone is a precursor of dihydrotestosterone, just as dehydroepiandrosterone (DHEA) is a precursor of testosterone. Neither testosterone nor DHEA can replace dihydrotestosterone.

In aging men and women, there is an overall lack of androgen production when dihydrotestosterone is low. Then the global production of anabolic hormones starts to decrease, although the nonsexual functions are, in part, spared.

Heavy testosterone treatments are dangerous for men with low testosterone (i.e., whose *production* of male hormones is almost nonexistent). In this condition, all arterial muscle structures have already been degenerating for decades, thus limiting life expectancy to eighty years on average.

As for women, they do not have an age-dependent treatment for androgens because this need is ignored and even prohibited by the pharmaceutical industry.

However, it is possible to compensate for the lack of anabolism at its inception. It is enough to take mesterolone, at the outset of the deficiency, depending on the biochemical dosage characteristics of each individual, which is around forty years of age and sometimes even before.

Mesterolone is not a potent anabolic. Therefore, it is scorned by the medical corps in the treatment of low testosterone syndrome in older men. In contrast, this medical condition would not even exist if correct prevention by mesterolone had been done forty years earlier.

Mesterolone is a weak anabolic, which gives it exceptional therapeutic quality. Its anabolic attributes are enough to maintain the networks of arterial muscle fibers to work throughout life. It is a hormone for a long, healthy life, a keystone.

In general, mesterolone is prescribed for a few months in men with a deficiency in androgen production. Women are excluded from treatment by the pharmaceutical industry, with the reasoning that the dosage of tablets sold is suitable for men only. The pharmaceutical industry has not yet realized the potential of mesterolone tablets for women. They would be quite simple to produce.

However, the prevention of arteriosclerosis must begin around age forty years, and sometimes even before, with daily doses taken throughout life. In my experience, three older people over age eighty—a woman and two men—were found to have a blood pressure of 12/8 and even 12/7.5 after several decades of continuous and preventive treatment with mesterolone [6]. This treatment is the prevention of high blood pressure after age forty, and the prevention of all disorders caused or aggravated by arteriosclerosis.

With monitoring of the production of dihydrotestosterone in the general framework of the overall output of androgens, it is possible to compensate for the deficiencies of anabolism.

Therefore, mesterolone should be the best-selling drug in the world because it would be beneficial for everyone [6].

13

Anemia

Red blood cells (RBCs) contain hemoglobin, a protein substance that contains iron and plays a crucial role in the transport of oxygen. The reduction of RBCs in the blood and of their hemoglobin content provokes anemia.

The main symptoms of anemia are paleness, tiredness, breathlessness and pulse acceleration, syncope, giddiness, and digestive disorders. Anemia can result from heavy bleeding (hemorrhage) or a disorder in the formation of RBCs resulting from infectious or toxic agents. RBCs also depend on specific hormones that stimulate their formation.

The number of RBCs in women varies between 3,500,000 and 5,500,000 per cubic millimeter of blood (standards can vary according to laboratories). Symptoms of anemia can appear below 3,500,000 RBCs per cubic millimeter of blood.

The "normal" number of globules is a statistical notion relating to the whole of the adult female population; however, each person is singular. Let us imagine that the ideal number of RBCs in a woman is 5,500,000 per cubic millimeter of blood. A laboratory result reporting 3,500,000 RBCs will be regarded as "normal" by the doctor, that is, located within a statistical average. Compared with the ideal number of RBCs for this same woman, however, she is missing two million RBCs per cubic millimeter of plasma, or 27.5 percent. It is consequently useful to know the number of RBCs at around age twenty, when the body is in full form, and to compare this number with the blood samples taken during aging. A drop of 10 to 20 percent in RBCs can decrease tissue oxygenation.

When the number of RBCs borders on 3,500,000, one can wonder whether the condition of anemia exists, with this average seeming to be "normal." The biological averages calculated with the whole of an older population are lowered because the physiological levels of young women become increasingly marginal in terms of "average." At the limit, young people, being a minority, would be regarded as "abnormal." It is necessary to provide further attention to this drift of statistical interpretation.

Medically, to impose this average on an overall population constitutes a severe and worse error—more, a fault. Each human being is singular and represents a vital force, worthy of greater respect.

The influence of male hormones on the formation of RBCs has been known for many years. Castration in rats produces a drop in male hormones and the appearance of anemia [1].

In 1956, Kennedy noted that women presenting with advanced breast cancer suffered from anemia. After giving them male hormones, the number of RBCs increased spectacularly [2,3].

Many diseases cause anemia. Treatment with male hormones is beneficial for many patients [4]. In 1981, Najean showed, in a series of 137 patients treated for more than two years, that anemia worsened with the stoppage of the administration of male hormones and improved when the treatment was reinstituted [5]. In laboratories today, one can study the effect of male hormones on stem cells of bone marrow put in cultures. These cells make RBCs, typically with male hormones [6].

Women with *androgenic menopausal disease* often present with a reduction in RBCs, which can be increased by taking male hormones.

In 2006, a study published in the *Archives of Internal Medicine* showed a high risk of anemia among men and women presenting with low testosterone levels. These scientific investigations were carried out by the Clinical Research Branch of the National Institute of Aging of Baltimore, in partnership with several scientific centers [7].

14

Viscous Blood, Embolisms, Thrombosis, Varicose Veins, and Hemorrhoids

Viscous Blood

The formation of a clot is caused by many factors that act successively to create a chain reaction, leading finally to the formation of fibrin, which is an insoluble fibrillary gel constituting the clot. Blood would coagulate if no factors were causing, at the same time, permanent lysis of the clot (fibrinolysis).

All in all, blood is composed of specific chemical factors that cause coagulation and chemical activators (e.g., antithrombin III) that ensure fluidity. The chemical reactions that start coagulation and those that cause fluidity are complex. The important thing is to know is that these forces are in permanent balance.

When factors of coagulation are missing, unverifiable hemorrhages sometimes occur. Hemophilia is well known. It is a hereditary disease characterized by a delay of coagulation and disproportionately prolonged hemorrhages that lack the tendency to stop spontaneously. In individuals with hemophilia, even the removal of a tooth constitutes a significant risk. Trauma can cause bleeding in the muscles or the articulations and can be fatal. Fortunately, hemophilia is an uncommon illness.

On the other hand, the excessive coagulation of blood is a widespread phenomenon after the age of sixty years. The factors of fluidity become unable to ensure the normal fluidity of the blood. Thick blood gives rise to thromboses and embolisms.

Thromboses

The formation of a clot in a blood vessel causes its occlusion. This can occur in an artery or a vein.

An arterial thrombosis develops at the wear points of arterial walls, caused by arteriosclerosis. The arteries of the extremities are most often reached, which can evolve into gangrene. Thrombosis from cerebral arteries has severe neurological consequences, such as paralysis.

A venous thrombosis comes from a slowing down of the bloodstream or uncontrolled coagulation forces. The phenomenon is already worrying when it develops in medium-caliber veins, but when it occurs in large blood vessels, it can be fatal.

Embolisms

The sudden obliteration of a vessel is a serious incident. It results from a clot that detaches from the heart's walls when there is a cardiac failure or from zones of excessive turbulence at arterial walls, arterial junctions, or atheromas. The abrupt obliteration of a large artery requires urgent surgery under the care of a surgeon who specializes in vascular techniques.

Cardiovascular disease is the primary source of thromboses and embolisms. Therefore, many patients permanently take anticoagulant medicines. They must check the fluidity of their blood with repeated blood examinations because these substances, to be active, must sufficiently lower the coagulation factors. Treatment with anticoagulants is not without risk. Beyond a critical point, a renal, gastric, or cerebral hemorrhage can occur.

The most used anticoagulants are heparin and dicoumarol. Heparin, used in intravenous injections, acts instantaneously. It inhibits the first and second stages of coagulation.

Dicoumarol taken orally works more slowly. It inhibits the K_1 vitamin necessary for the first stage of clotting. Patients who receive this treatment must permanently supervise their prothrombin times, which must range between 20 and 30 percent. Below that, there is a risk of bleeding.

Dicoumarol prevents blood from coagulating but does not cause the dissolution of the clot, which is done by other molecules. Thick blood results from an incapacity of fluidity factors to create the clot lysis. Patients having thromboembolic vascular disorders present with a defect of fibrinolysis.

Male Hormones Are Natural Blood Thinners

In 1988, Bonithon-Kopp and colleagues [1] showed that low plasma testosterone levels were associated with a hypercoagulability of the blood. The same year, Caron and colleagues [2] confirmed that fibrinolysis represents an essential system against the development of venous and arterial thromboses and is influenced favorably by male hormones. Other authors prescribed male hormones to thin the blood of patients suffering from vascular disorders [3,4]. By managing male hormones, the blood becomes thin as a result of the increase in the production of antithrombin III (a thinning factor). When treatment is interrupted, the blood becomes thick again because of the reduction of antithrombin III production. Blood once again becomes fluid with the resumption of androgens.

In conclusion, male hormones constitute natural factors of blood fluidity by stimulating the production of antithrombin III. Their administration does not present a danger of bleeding, contrary to anticoagulants. The World Health Organization recommends the treatment of thromboembolic cardiovascular diseases with testosterone [5].

Antithrombin (also called *antithrombin III* or *AT III*) belongs to the class of substances that are inhibitors of coagulation. A deficit in antithrombin predisposes to thromboses.

In 2009, a study showed that testosterone administration increased fluidity factors in people with diabetes with foot ulcers [6].

Varicose Veins and Hemorrhoids

Heavy Legs

Varicose veins develop with age, especially in the legs. Superficial veins are dilated, irregular, tortuous, and unaesthetic in appearance. After a prolonged upright position, they cause a feeling of having "heavy legs," which is accentuated gradually until the day's end. The feet are inflated by edema.

Varicose veins can also be the consequence of compression of the venous network. This phenomenon is rare in men. In women, who are more predisposed to develop varicose veins, venous dilations of the legs can appear during pregnancy. They become more frequent with obesity and age. Varicose veins can become complicated by varicose phlebitis and ulcers.

Phlebitis is an inflammation of the venous walls. It causes pulmonary embolisms in 5 to 6 percent of cases. Pulmonary embolism represents a significant cause of mortality and results in more than fifty thousand deaths in the United States each year. Pulmonary embolism is fatal in only 10 percent of cases; thus, one can estimate the annual number of pulmonary embolisms in the US as more than five hundred thousand.

A varicose ulcer is significant ulceration of the leg, usually caused by a chronic venous insufficiency. The loss of skin substance is sometimes the result of minor trauma, a common cutaneous infection, or the thrombosis of a dilated vein. Varicose ulcers are difficult to cure.

Hemorrhoids

Varicose veins of anus and rectum create venous tumors called *hemorrhoids*. Like all varicose veins, they can cause inflammation and painful thromboses. External hemorrhoids are located below the anal sphincter and are visible to the naked eye. Internal hemorrhoids, located above the anal sphincter, are viewable by anoscopy.

Except for the compression phenomena, medical books do not explain why venous walls can be weak in humans.

Veins, like the arteries, consist of elastic tissues. After having irrigated organs, blood returns to the heart through the venous network. Initially, small venules collect blood and then increasingly larger veins. The venules continue in the muscular veins of the extremities and internal organs. Some of these veins are strengthened and constitute a system of pumps, which propel blood toward the heart, such as the pelvic veins, the large veins of the lower extremities, and the large vena cava.

A lack of male hormones automatically causes the same regressive transformations as those observed in the musculature of arterial walls.

The smooth muscles degenerate replaced by rigid fibrous tissue. Also, the other elastic components lose their elasticity. These degenerative transformations compromise the propulsion of blood. The return of blood toward the heart is impaired. An excess of coagulation is responsible for unexplained phlebitis [7] and certain leg ulcers [8].

Bennet and colleagues [9] showed, in 1987, that venous stagnation tends to form clots in patients having a lack of male hormones. This tendency toward thrombosis normalized after three months' treatment with dihydrotestosterone, managed as a cutaneous gel at a rate of 125 milligrams per day.

Male hormones are necessary for the flexibility of venous walls and to ensure blood fluidity.

15

Hypertension: A Worldwide Disease

According to the World Health Organization (WHO), cardiovascular diseases were responsible for approximately 17 million deaths in the world in 2008—that is to say, nearly a third of the total mortality rate. Of this, 9.4 million deaths a year are caused by complications of hypertension (high blood pressure). Hypertension is responsible for at least 45 percent of deaths from cardiac diseases and 51 percent of deaths from strokes.

In 2016, hypertension affected nearly one-third of US residents aged 18 years or older (approximately 75 million persons), and in roughly half of adults with hypertension (almost 35 million persons), it is uncontrolled. Among these 35 million US residents with unchecked hypertension, 33 percent (11.5 million persons) are not aware of their hypertension, and 20 percent (7 million persons) are aware of their hypertension but are not treated. Approximately 47 percent (16.1 million persons) are aware of their hypertension and being treated for it, but treatment (by medication and lifestyle modification) is not adequately controlling their blood pressure [1].

Arterial hypertension is one of the most critical problems concerning public health in the world. Its insidious development over the years makes it even more dangerous because it does not appear with alarming symptoms at the beginning. When they occur, hypertension is already very advanced. Hypertension is a silent assassin. Ideal blood pressure is twelve centimeters of mercury for the maximum pressure and eight centimeters of mercury for the minimum pressure [2]. The continual rise in centimeters of mercury, over one or two pressure readings, means that the tension is too high. The cardiovascular mortality rate rises immediately. Minimal tension with nine centimeters of mercury is already a bad sign. When the maximum pressure exceeds 15.8, cardiovascular risk is multiplied by 2.5. A blood pressure of 14/9 calls for immediate therapeutic measures.

The frequency of arterial hypertension is impressive. Framingham, quoted by Williams and Braunwald in *Harrison's Principles of Internal Medicine* in 1989 [3], showed in a population of white people living in suburbs that 20 percent of the subjects had blood pressures higher than 16/9.5, whereas 50 percent of them had arterial pressure of 14/9.

These same authors specify that the cause of arterial hypertension is unknown in most cases. Doctors call this type of hypertension *essential* or *idiopathic*, which simply means the etiology is unknown. Classically, it is considered a hereditary condition. Essential hypertension represents 90 percent of arterial hypertension cases.

In 2017, new guidelines from the American Heart Association, the American College of Cardiology, and nine other health organizations lowered the numbers for the diagnosis of hypertension to 130/80 millimeters of mercury (mm Hg) and higher for all adults. The previous guidelines set the threshold at 140/90 mm Hg for people younger than age sixty-five- and 150/80 mm Hg for those aged sixty-five and older. Now, 70 to 79 percent of men aged fifty-five and older have hypertension. That includes many men whose blood pressure had previously been considered healthy [4].

In April 2018, Harvard Health Publishing of the Harvard Medical School defined new blood pressure guidelines. The definition of high blood pressure has tightened. Here is what you need to know (table 14).

Blood Pressure Categories			
Blood Pressure	Systolic mm Hg (Upper Number)		Systolic mm Hg (Lower Number)
Normal	Less than 120	and	Less than 80
Elevated	120–129	and	Less than 80
Hypertension stage 1	130–139	or	80-89
Hypertension stage 2	**140 or higher**	**or**	**90 or higher**
Hypertensive crisis	**Higher than 180**	**and**	**Higher than 120**

Table 14

The maximum and minimum arterial pressures are the expressions of the variations of pressure exerted via blood on the walls of a closed elastic circuit. These pressures are caused by two engines that take turns: the cardiac muscle and the musculature of the arteries.

The cardiac contraction is responsible for the maximal arterial pressure caused by the shock of the blood wave on the walls of large arteries, transmitting the stream in the arterial system.

The contraction of the arterial muscles takes over, between two cardiac contractions, to ensure the continuity of the propulsion of the blood wave in the tiny arteries (small arteries). It causes the minimum pressure. If this secondary engine did not exist, the blood pressure would fall to zero between two pulsations from the heart.

Blood circulates permanently in the organs because of the successive contractions of these two powerful engines, which propel blood in the tiny arteries and the capillaries. They are the most elementary blood vessels, the last ramifications of the circulatory system, which connect small arteries and venules. This final vascular network does not have an engine; blood circulates there continuously because of the cardiac and arterial propulsion, constituting the peripheral resistance of the vascular system.

The cardiac pump must provide an extra effort to propel blood when arterial resistance increases in the large arteries: the maximum pressure rises, and heart work increases by 40 to 50 percent. The muscular pump of the arteries must also provide an extra effort to propel the blood wave in the network of small arteries, which increases resistance; the minimum pressure thus rises.

Untreated hypertension is associated with a reduction in the life span of about ten to twenty years.

A combination of factors causes an increase in blood pressure with age. They are the rigidity of the arterial walls, the increase in peripheral resistance, and the high viscosity of the blood. For the system to work well, all components must be intact, which is generally the case at twenty years of age.

The origin of essential hypertension is the consequence of the degeneration of the system. The rigidity of the arterial walls and an increase in peripheral resistance are the most degenerative factors.

The elasticity of arterial walls decreases because of arteriosclerosis and atheroma. These phenomena develop with age according to the reduction in the secretion of male hormones. It is enough to examine the small arteries of the retina; their aspects are representative of that of cerebral arteries and the arterial system in general.

The increase in peripheral resistance involves an unbearable cardiac overload. The mass to irrigate is the resistance. How does this mass increase? The brain volume does not increase, nor does the size of other organs. What, then, can increase the mass of the human body with time? Fat. It settles everywhere in the body. In man, it is stored mainly in the belly, around the intestines. One often finds there ten to twenty useless kilos. Fat is a living tissue nourished by the last ends of the arterial network, which builds up there.

Additional resistance in the arterial system increases according to the increase in the fatty mass. It is because of this factor that it is necessary to act from the first extra kilo.

We saw in chapter 10 how fat tissue develops from a lack of male hormones and overeating. A blood pressure of 12/8 at twenty years of age accompanies a relatively low weight. If you suffer from essential hypertension, it is necessary to go back to the weight you were at age twenty. It is entirely possible.

Hypercoagulability is also the result of the lack of male hormones. More viscous blood increases the force necessary for the propulsion of the blood wave.

Traditional hypertension treatment uses substances that act on the nervous system of muscular arteries by causing their relaxation. Beta-blocker drugs, which block the action of nervous fibers causing arterial contraction, are useful but treat only the symptom and not the cause of hypertension. Although the blood pressure drops, beta-blocker drugs protect the heart but make the blood pressure drop at the periphery. For example, the arteries of the penis of a hypertensive man are part of the final network. The taking of beta-blockers makes the pressure in the penis fall, causing impotence. The same applies to the ultimate arterial system and all organs; they will suffer from a lack of irrigation.

It is possible, in many cases, to be released from the beta-blocker treatment by paying particular attention to the control of weight and by decreasing the sclerosis of arteries with male hormones. This treatment is a correct approach from the appearance of the first symptoms. It constitutes a significant preventive measure for hypertension. When the whole of the arterial system becomes rigid, it is still possible to improve the vascular state, but many lesions will have become irreversible.

Hypertension causes the appearance of all kinds of mechanisms and pathological vicious circles that worsen arterial hypertension. They are responsible for many strokes and dramatic arterial ruptures.

At the time of the 2013 World Health Day, the WHO published a remarkable world panorama of hypertension. It stated, "The risk of hypertension increases with age because of the hardening of the blood vessels, although the aging of the latter can be slowed down by the adoption of healthy lifestyles, including a balanced diet and a reduction in the consumption of salt."

Certain people manage to limit their blood pressure by changing their lifestyles by, for example, stopping tobacco use, eating healthily, getting regular physical exercise, and avoiding the harmful use of alcohol. All adults should control their blood pressure. If it rises, they must consult a health professional.

The lack of testosterone responsible for arteriosclerosis is the leading cause of essential arterial hypertension in women, who need individual attention. For technical reasons, mesterolone is the right treatment, not testosterone (chapter 31).

Variations in Blood Pressure, in Centimeters of Mercury, According to Age, in 250,000 Americans in Good Health		
Age	Maximum Pressure	Minimum Pressure
10	10.3	7
15	11.3	7.5
20	**12**	**8**
25	12.2	8.1
30	12.3	8.2
35	12.4	8.3
40	12.6	8.4
45	12.8	8.5
50	13	8.6
55	13.2	8.7
60	13.5	8.9

Table 15

Statistics from Hunter quoted by Best and Taylor [2].

Fibrous tissue replaces arterial muscle, degenerating fibers. In the beginning, only visible at the microscopic level, that constitutes a dynamic obstacle to blood flow in the absence of an arterial narrowing that would be seen by the eye (chapter 12).

Essential hypertension represents 90 percent of arterial hypertension cases that are the result of arteriosclerosis. The cause of arteriosclerosis is the progressive atrophy of arterial muscle fibers due to a lack of anabolic hormones from the age of twenty-five years.

The blood pressure of 12/8 is normal. It is the case at age twenty.

Table 15 shows the progressive elevation of blood pressure after age twenty. It is remarkable to note that at age twenty-five, blood pressure already increases moderately. From age twenty-five to sixty, the maximum and minimum pressures increase continually with years.

Hypertension intensifying with age in the whole of a population [2] begs the question about an essential cause that accentuates its effects with time.

At age twenty-five, the human being is in top form, with average quantities of anabolic hormones produced by the body. From age twenty-five on, the production of male hormones decreases in parallel to the increase in blood pressure. This phenomenon is the cause of arteriosclerosis.

16

Coronary Disease and Heart Infarct

Cardiac Diseases and Atheroma

Angina pectoris is the expression of a temporary reduction in the oxygenation of the cardiac muscle.

The work of the heart requires a permanent oxygen contribution, transported by the blood that circulates in the arteries of the heart, the coronary arteries. There are two. One irrigates the anterior wall; the other irrigates the posterior wall of the heart. These two arteries meet in the cardiac muscle.

The most frequent cause of angina pectoris in a woman with menopausal disease is atherosclerosis of the coronary arteries, in which fatty deposits decrease the diameter of the principal or secondary arteries in one or more places.

Emotional factors can also cause a crisis of angina pectoris by producing an intense spasm of the heart's arteries, causing insufficient irrigation of the cardiac muscle.

The contribution of oxygenated blood decreases more, especially in narrowed arteries. In the beginning, reduced physical activity does not start the crisis. The insufficiency of blood irrigation appears during a physical effort, which causes a precordial pain. The blood is unable to ensure sufficient oxygenation of the heart during this extra work. The crisis occurs, for example, while running to catch the train or the bus.

When the diameter of the artery is reduced by more than 80 percent, the arterial flow is insufficient at rest. Crises can occur at any time, even in bed. A more severe reduction of the arterial gauge causes dramatic heart diseases like myocardial infarction. A tight contracting of the anterior coronary artery has a mortality rate of 15 percent per year.

Electrocardiograms show characteristic signs when the contracting of the heart's arteries is problematic. At rest, these modifications are not always manifest when the arteries moderately narrowed. In this case, electrocardiogram modifications are visible by a stress test. The stress test is performed on a bicycle, under the control of a cardiologist.

The localization of the arterial narrowing is put in evidence by the coronary angiography (radiographs of heart arteries). A catheter, introduced into a large artery of the leg, goes up toward the heart and selectively penetrates the coronary artery to inject a contrast medium there.

Cardiovascular mortality is in direct correlation with the evolution of atheroma deposits in the heart's arteries. We saw in chapter 9 how metabolic trouble because of fats and cholesterol in the metabolism increases this evolution. The rise in fats (triglycerides) in the blood significantly increases the risk of narrowing of the heart arteries. The increase in "bad" cholesterol (low-density lipoprotein [LDL] cholesterol) is in correlation with coronary insufficiency.

Studies have shown the crucial role of "good" cholesterol (high-density lipoprotein [HDL] cholesterol) in the prevention of coronary disease. Cholesterol is transported in the blood current by specific proteins (HDLs) whose principal function is to collect cholesterol in several sites and carry it toward the liver, where it is degraded and excreted in the bile. HDL proteins are, all in all, the "street sweepers" of cholesterol.

The Framingham Heart Study showed that for both men and women, an HDL cholesterol level of higher than fifty-two milligrams per hundred cubic centimeters of plasma constitutes a protective factor against the risk of coronary insufficiency [1].

Foods rich in animal fats cause a rise in harmful fats in the blood and determine the appearance of cardiovascular disease.

On the other hand, populations that stick to a vegetarian diet that is low in fats are less predisposed to cardiovascular diseases. The Bantu vegetarians, for example, experienced a rise in blood cholesterol after having left the rural areas for the city and having modified their dietary habits by eating Western food.

A woman with coronary insufficiency must reexamine her lifestyle by controlling her food intake and her physical activity. She must avoid smoking and eliminate any causes of stress.

High Rate	Correlation with Coronary Insufficiency
Total cholesterol	+
LDL cholesterol	+
Triglycerides	+
HDL cholesterol	–

Table 16

Testosterone Deficit and Cardiac Diseases

Deficits in male hormones and disturbances in their metabolism have been correlated with cardiac disease for about fifty years, and the first treatments with testosterone date back to that time.

Coronary Insufficiency

Angina pectoris is a transitory pain felt at the level of the heart. Men account for 80 percent of cases beyond age fifty and a higher percentage before this age. The pain is a discomfort in the chest, where it appears like a heaviness, a feeling of oppression or smothering, or an impression of squeezing or compression. The intensity of this discomfort is generally variable and lasts from one to five minutes. The pain can be perceived in the left shoulder and the arms.

The narrowing of coronary arteries is in correlation with the disturbance of sex hormones. This lesser-known reality is, however, essential. Coronary insufficiency appears with the disruption of sex hormone levels. The male hormones, testosterone and dihydrotestosterone, are in perpetual balance with the female hormone, estradiol, in women.

The heart functions well with the right levels of male hormones and when female hormones do not exceed an ideal level. The excess of female hormones neutralizes male hormones.

Several studies have shown a correlation between coronary insufficiency and the existence, on the one hand, of a low testosterone level and, on the other hand, a high level of female hormones. The levels of male and female hormones can be simultaneously disturbed. Insufficient production of dihydrotestosterone corresponds to coronary insufficiency (table 17).

The traditional treatment of coronary insufficiency does not consider the crucial role of male hormones. Individual doctors, however, have understood it and treated heart cases successfully with male hormones.

In 1946, Lesser published a five-year study on 101 patients suffering from angina pectoris who were treated with testosterone propionate [2]. There were ninety-two men and eight women, from thirty-four to seventy-seven years old.

Symptoms improved in ninety-one percent of cases for periods varying between two and thirty-four months. Most patients received, twice per week, twenty-five milligrams of hormones by intramuscular injections over two weeks, followed by a weekly dose of twenty-five milligrams.

Hormone	Plasma Level	Correlation with Coronary Insufficiency
Total testosterone	Low	+
Free testosterone	Low	+
Dihydrotestosterone	Low	+
Estradiol	Raised	+

Table 17

A reference group of patients having received sesame oil injections not containing hormones did not present any improvement of the painful symptoms. The patients treated with testosterone reacted favorably to the treatment and did not show any undesirable effects.

Four patients were given stress tests before and during the hormonal therapy to measure the improvement of their cardiac states objectively. Each one of them was able to expend more effort during the hormonal treatment compared with their former conditions, and the duration of painful heart attacks shortened. In each case, subjective improvement preceded objective measurements of improved cardiac work.

An insufficiency of the secretion of male sex hormones intervenes decisively in a disordered state of metabolism of sugars, fats, and cholesterol. This lack is responsible for arteriosclerosis and atheroma. The correlation of the insufficiency of hormonal secretion with coronary insufficiency is a reality.

Heart Infarct

Until the eighteenth century, cardiac diseases were unknown and even denied. Diderot affirms in his *Encyclopedia* that heart diseases were uncommon.

It was only during the twentieth century, especially after 1940, that heart disease became the focus of attention, with coronary syndromes constituting a disaster in industrialized countries.

Narrowed arteries of the heart do not flood certain parts of the cardiac muscle, which then become necrotic, sometimes in a dramatic way.

The heart was, from time immemorial, regarded as the center of the human. It became the emblem of courage, intelligence, and friendship. In a word, the heart symbolizes love. More prosaically, the heart is a muscle—an automatic muscle, yes, but before all, a muscle. To contract, it needs, like the skeletal muscle, the force of contractile proteins and fuel—glycogen, which is fundamental.

The chemistry of cardiac muscle contraction depends on the action of male hormones. They are specific receptors for testosterone in the muscle fibers of a rat's heart [3,4]. Other experiments have shown an increase in actinomyosin content in cardiac muscle with testosterone administration [5]. This substance reinforces the specific contractile elements.

Older heart disease sufferers have been advised to take all kinds of regulating drugs for their heart problems. Do they know that an essential "food" for the heart, testosterone, is missing? Male hormones reinforce the muscular contraction of cardiac muscle, just as they reinforce the actions of the other muscular tissues. Taking androgens improves the work of the insufficient or degenerated heart.

In 1996, Dominique Simon (of unit 21 of the INSERM [the French National Institute of Health and Medical Research]), Khalil Nahoul, and their collaborators confirmed the favorable impact of testosterone on cardiovascular risk factors. This study, known as the Telecom Study [6], proceeded over eight years and compared the parameters of cardiovascular risk (HDL cholesterol, LDL cholesterol, triglycerides, blood sugar, and so on) of two groups of men.

The first group, whose blood testosterone levels remained stable for eight years, did not show any increase in vascular risk for this period. The second group, whose blood testosterone levels decreased for this period, showed a significant increase in cardiovascular risk [6].

Androgen hormones, well proportioned, reduce cholesterol levels naturally. In this case, one can observe the fall of the good cholesterol (HDL cholesterol) in the blood. In 2012, a study of the University of Washington School of Medicine in Seattle showed that this reduction corresponds to an accelerated transport of HDL cholesterol [7].

In the same year, researchers in the Cardiovascular Department of Medicine at the University of Harbin in China showed an interesting fact in castrated rats. Those animals had a heart infarct following the binding of a coronary artery. The hormonal replacement of testosterone caused the appearance of new blood vessels [8].

In 2010, researchers from the Department of Endocrinology, Max Planck Institute of Psychiatry, Munich, Germany, concluded that low baseline testosterone in women is associated with increased all-cause mortality and cardiovascular events, independent of traditional risk factors [9].

Myocardial infarction is the final expression of a morbid process generated by the lack of energy substances necessary to the cardiac muscle, worsened by degeneration of the coronary arteries.

Male hormones thin the blood and increase the contractile force of the cardiac muscle. They support healing by stimulation of protein synthesis and cause revascularization of the heart.

17

Stiffness, Limitation of Movement, Slipped Discs, and Degenerative Joint Disease

With age, stiffness occurs when the ligaments, tendons, and fibrous tissues of the body retract.

Causes of Degenerative Joint Disease

It is necessary to know some elements of the nature and biochemistry of conjunctive tissues. These tissues occupy the intervals between the organs and constitute the details of an organ. They are components of mechanical support and framing. They consist of cells and fibers that "bathe" in a kind of gel (fundamental substance) made up of specialized molecules. It is through conjunctive tissue that nutritive molecules and oxygen arrive in the organism's cells.

Fibrocytes, the conjunctive cells, generate fibers. The most well-known are the collagenous fibers. They meet in almost all conjunctive tissues and consist of subunits situated outside of the cells that formed them. The *collagenous* (in French, from *colle* and *gene*) qualifier comes from the name of the proteins that constitute these fibers. They are transformed into gelatin by heat.

The high resistance of collagen to traction confers the solidity of conjunctive tissues.

The tangle of fibers adapts perfectly to the structures that surround specific tissues. Collagenous fibers constitute the essence of ligament and tendon structures, perhaps the best known being the Achilles tendon. Inserted on the heel's bone, it is prone to injuries and ruptures during excessive physical effort.

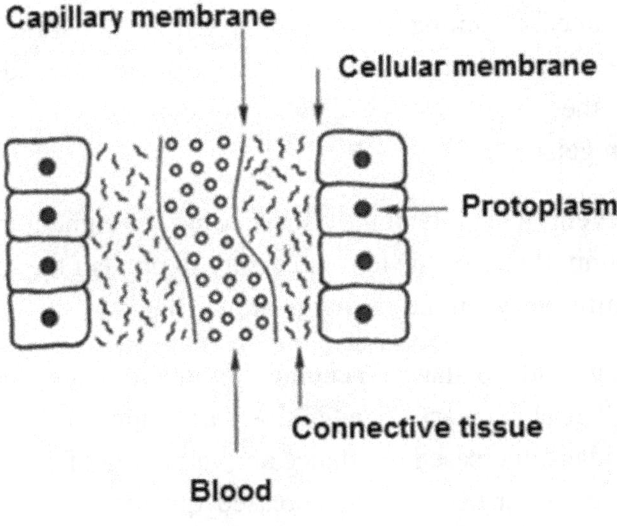

Fig. 23

Diagram of the barrier to enter blood and tissues.

After Sobel and Marmorston [4].

Collagenous fibers constitute the essence of ligament and tendon structures, perhaps the best known being the Achilles tendon. Inserted on the heel's bone, it is prone to injuries and ruptures during excessive physical effort.

Collagenous proteins have a probable lifetime of several years, but the measurement is difficult. In the event of wounds, specialized cells make new fibers to fill the gap, constituting scar tissue.

Ligaments and tendons retract with age. To pick up a paper from the ground or to put on a coat becomes an increasingly hard operation.

Thus, the cells of the organism age, but the matter that surrounds and supports cells ages too. This phenomenon was shown by the famous experiments of Hungarian physiologist Fritz Verzar. He suspended collagen filaments coming from a rat's tail in a bain-marie at a temperature from thirty-seven to forty degrees. Under these conditions, the fibers shortened, the proteins of collagen being denatured in gelatin.

One can prevent the shortening by suspending a weight at the end of fibers. The importance of the load necessary to prevent the shortening is more significant when the animal is old [1,2].

As we grow old, collagen becomes more resistant instead of weakening. The elementary collagen fibers are connected to others by chemical bridges. Increased resistance and retraction of collagen with age are the consequences of an increased quantity of bridges or a change in their chemical nature.

Glucose has the property of being fixed on all proteins. The excessive presence of glucose in the body accentuates the structural transformation of healthy collagen into rigid. It is the billions of glucose molecules that "stick" chemically elementary collagen fibers between them [3]. All conditions that abnormally raise blood glucose cause the abnormal bridging of collagen. Male hormones play a crucial role in lowering the level of blood glucose (see chapter 8).

Insufficient secretion of male hormones causes a tendency toward increased blood sugar, itself responsible for the abnormal collagen bridging, which causes retraction of ligaments and tendons. For this reason, while being "too sweetened," the woman with *androgenic menopausal disease* becomes stiff.

Rigid collagenous fibers and cells bathe in a gelatinous substance. This gel constitutes an obligatory method for the transport of nutritive molecules and oxygen in cells. With age, the composition of this extracellular gel deteriorates, compromising the nutrition of cellular compartments.

The scarcity of the gelatinous substance is a consequence of the insufficiency of the secretion of male hormones. This phenomenon was shown in 1958 by Sobel and Marmorston from the Institute for Medical Research, Cedars of Lebanon Hospital, and the Department of Biochemistry and Nutrition and the Department of Medicine, University of Southern California, Los Angeles, California [4].

Hand Pains

Fibrosis and retraction of the wrist's ligaments can compress the nerves that arrive at the hand. Under these conditions, the median nerve can be compacted, causing pains in the thumb, the index finger, or the middle finger. Specialized surgery that decompresses nerves eliminates the pain.

Finger Retractions

Retraction of the superficial fascia, which covers the palm, is particularly spectacular. The fingers become curled up and immobilized in this position. To correct this infirmity, traditional treatment resorts to a specialized surgery that treats the consequence of the disease and not the cause. The operation does not prevent repetition. Retraction of the hand's ligaments depends on the hormonal balance, which modifies the composition of fibrous tissue and causes the contraction of the tiny arteries.

As always, it is necessary to act from the beginning of the disease, correcting what it might lead to without waiting for curled fingers. A lack of male hormones induces a whole series of biochemical reactions that causes the degeneration of tissues. However, further research will be needed in this field.

Diseases of aging are caused in men and women when insufficient production of androgens is confirmed by low levels of androgens (see chapter 5) [5].

Slipped Discs

Vertebrae are separated by intervertebral discs, which cushion the impact of shocks on the vertebrae. The intervertebral disc degenerates from a lack of male hormones and becomes thin. The overlying and underlying vertebrae move toward each other, causing a vertebral "pinching" at the origin of often intolerable pain caused by excessive pressure of the vertebrae on the nerves that leave the spinal column. This widespread phenomenon in women with androgenic menopausal disease usually requires surgery to decompress the crushed nerves. The supervening of a first slipped disc in a woman with androgenic illness of menopause is a severe symptom.

This degeneration announces other degenerations of her joint articulations and ligaments. Then it is the totality of her body that degenerates as a result of a lack of male hormones that have the biological property of rebuilding intervertebral ligaments, discs, and articulations.

When the secretion of male hormones is not enough, the recurrence of slipped discs is the rule, leading to new surgeries.

The joint articulations degenerate on one side or both sides. Being overweight worsens the excessive pressure on afflicted articulations, thus delaying the healing of any surgical procedure. Attempts at slimming decrease the mass and the muscular force, whatever the regime, causing a functional overload of the affected and operated-on articulations. The slimming diet will have better results with the administration of male hormones, which decrease fat and improve the mass and the muscular force (chapters 10 and 11).

The situation also becomes complicated by the infection of surgically treated articulations in a woman with androgenic menopausal disease because her immune system can be defective (chapter 24).

Cascading catastrophes lead to multiple surgical procedures, which could be avoided by the prevention of degeneration with male hormones.

The biological rebuilding of discs, ligaments, and articulations could take several years if hormonal treatment was ignored and replaced by successive surgical procedures. Hormonal therapy can be lifesaving.

Degenerative Joint Disease or Osteoarthritis

Osteoarthritis is a degenerative disease of the joint articulations. All are involved, but those used for support are particularly predisposed.

Osteoarthritis is frequent in women after age forty-five and becomes more common as the age is advanced. It is practically constant after age seventy-five.

Movement confers to women their physical freedom and autonomy, essential to their survival. Mobility characterizes a particular functional entity: the articulation. The support and slip functions are facilitated by the cartilage that covers the two osseous ends linked by a capsule and ligaments. The joining capsule is lined inside by a special membrane, the synovial membrane, which secretes a lubricating liquid, synovia. Muscles inserted on both sides of osseous ends constitute the engine of articulation.

This functional entity is nourished by an arterial network, which ends in small arteries.

In the beginning, osteoarthritis appears as a limitation of movements. Pains clear up in the morning and disappear during the day. At this stage, the articulation does not show a clinical sign. Gradually, the motion becomes more limited because of the retraction and rigidity of ligaments, which form calcium and make crackling noises. While turning the head, for example, one perceives small cracklings in the neck.

This stage is already significant. It is here that it is necessary to act—quickly. The diagnosis is based primarily on radiographs that do not show anything. Of the four articular structures—the bone, the synovial membrane, the joint capsule, and the cartilage—only bones are visible on radiographs. The other structures are radiotransparent. Moreover, to appreciate a modification of the skeletal structure, one needs to know the essential variation of its calcium load. It is only when calcium loss reaches approximately 30 percent that one can detect an osseous decalcification with radiographs.

After many months and many years, the diagnosis of osteoarthritis finally becomes visible on radiographs. Articulation degeneration appears through cartilage destruction and the approach of the bony end. One feels articular pinching. The calcified ligaments and the joint capsule are visible around the articulation. Finally, skeletal ends, overloaded with calcium, are sometimes welded together, immobilizing the bones. Everyone knows a grandmother or grandfather with osteoarthritis. It usually began at age forty and was never cured. At present, nothing is done to prevent this degenerative phenomenon that ultimately strikes all older women.

All articulations undergo the same fate. The degenerative aspects are marked in the knee, hip, spinal column, and shoulder, which do more work.

Knee osteoarthritis appears as pain when going up and down staircases. The knee inflates, and the kneecap immobilizes. When articulation is completely blocked, one can remove the joint through surgery and replace it with an artificial knee. Knee osteoarthritis is an important topic because it affects the quality of life of millions of people. Women typically present with more advanced stages and more disability than men [6].

The prevalence of hip osteoarthritis is higher among men younger than age fifty years, whereas women have the highest incidence after age fifty years because of postmenopausal changes. It strikes both hips in 20 percent of cases. Pains while walking are perceived in the groin, the buttocks, the thigh, and the knee, which are calmed at rest. The articulation worsens gradually. The head of the femur, formerly round, is flattened into the shape of a "coach buffer." The bony cavity in which it is encased is overloaded with calcium and develops excrescences, immobilizing the articulation completely. The gait becomes lame. It is challenging to rise when from a seated position. Consequently, the muscles that surround the articulation degenerate in turn, producing a trailing gait.

That is no problem, traditional medicine will say; surgery is there to remove the affected articulation and replace it with a prosthesis. Unfortunately, the results are not definitive because the condition of the bone around the prosthesis worsens again. Many women undergo multiple replacements of hip prostheses, increasing the number of complicated and hazardous surgical procedures.

Vertebral osteoarthritis reaches the cervical, dorsal, or lumbar segment of the spinal column. One notes the calcareous overload of ligaments and osseous excrescences ("parrots' nozzles"). The collapse of the vertebrae causes pinching of the nerves that leave the spinal column, sometimes causing intolerable pain. That is no problem either; traditional medicine might say, surgery is there to decompress the wedged nerve. But surgery is not definitive. The bony substance worsens again, causing recurrence at the operated site or above or below it.

The cervical column and the lumbar column are reached first for mechanical reasons.

Osteoarthritis of the cervical column causes pain in the nape, sometimes radiating to the arm.

The compression of particular nerve roots causes headaches, giddiness, eye or auditory troubles, and pain in the face. The mobilization of the neck is limited and causes crackling.

Osteoarthritis of the dorsal column is rarer. The pinching of the nerves causes intercostal pain.

Lumbar osteoarthritis is widespread. It appears, in the beginning, after a little physical effort, starting an excruciating crisis of lumbago. The spasm of lumbar muscles immobilizes the patient for a few hours to a few days. This benign incident recurs.

Pain also radiates to the thighs and buttocks and the testicles in men. The compression of the sciatic nerve is particularly painful. It begins in the lumbar area, is propagated in the outer face of the leg, and finishes in the big toe. At an advanced stage, pain becomes permanent and prohibits the slightest efforts at movement.

Many causes of osteoarthritis are known. They all lead to the destruction of the cartilage, the genuine shock absorber of articulation. With time, the cartilage wears out like the shock absorbers of a car for all kinds of reasons.

Generally, the causes reside, on the one hand, in mechanical disorders of articulation (poorly assembled shock absorbers or having received an excessive shock) and, on the other hand, in structural disorders of the articulation itself (shock absorbers of poor quality).

Aging contributes to the development of hip osteoarthritis, mainly because of the inability to correctly define an underlying anatomic abnormality or specific disease process leading to the degenerative process [7]. Osteoarthritis of unknown origin accounts for 50 percent of the cases, gradually destroying the whole articular system. Medical books speak about *primitive osteoarthritis* to indicate osteoarthritis of unknown origin, which means nothing in terms of prevention and treatment.

One can wonder about a general cause that worsens with age.

The traditional treatment of osteoarthritis of unknown origin is primarily symptomatic and relates to its consequences. Pain can be relieved by aspirin. Anti-inflammatory drugs are not without disadvantages. They can cause bleeding or disorders of blood composition. Doctors sometimes inject cortisone around or in the articulation to reduce inflammation. These infiltrations must be made judiciously and not repeated too often.

Failure of these treatments gives way to osteopathy or manual therapy, which free the articulations and are helpful for the patient—temporarily. Lastly, in cases where other options have failed, surgery briskly replaces the completely worn joints.

Treatment of Degenerative Joint Disease with Male Hormones

My attention was very often drawn, during hormonal treatments for sexual insufficiency, to the reflections of patients who announced to me the disappearance of their shoulder, knee, or finger pain. "It is strange; my pains disappeared," they said.

At first, I did not attach importance to these comments. However, the repetition of these surprising testimonies eventually convinced me: male hormones act on osteoarthritis and prevent its development independently of any other factor. While reflecting, I realized that this fact is not astonishing for two essential reasons.

The first reason concerns the vascularization of the articulations. They are tiny arteries, without which neither oxygen nor nutritive substances can arrive at the specialized cells.

The cartilage does not contain small arteries; it is nourished by imbibition, starting from the articular liquid secreted by the synovial membrane, or by diffusion, beginning from the end of the bone where they branch and ending with the smallest arteries.

The small arteries degenerate when arteriosclerosis develops. We saw that arteriosclerosis develops more vigorously when male hormones are insufficient. Consequently, the secretion of the articular liquid will be compromised.

The second reason concerns the cartilage, consisting mostly of a fundamental substance that confers elasticity and resistance to an organism. One also finds collagenous fibers. Specialized cells of the cartilage make these protein structures. They constitute a living tissue that requires continuous maintenance. When male hormones are insufficient, the proteins' synthesis is compromised, and the cartilage degenerates.

These two essential consequences of the lack of male hormones seriously compromise the structures of all articulations. Osteoarthritis worsens even more in a woman with an excess of weight.

Many osteoarthritis cases of unknown origin are the consequence of arteriosclerosis of the tiny arteries of articulations. At the same time, the insufficiency of male hormone secretion provokes the degeneration of the articular cartilage. Prevention of osteoarthritis in time with mesterolone, in association with dieting, is a possible solution. When destroyed, however, articulations need conventional treatment.

18

Fragile Bones

Like all support tissues in general, bone tissue consists of specialized cells, fibers, and a fundamental substance. The bones collect mineral salts, especially calcic salts, which give its rigidity and its consistency.

Bone tissue has mechanical functions of support or protection. The pressure resistance of compact bone tissue is fifteen kilos per square millimeter. Moreover, the bone resists inflection and presents a certain degree of elasticity.

The bone is also a chemical tank. Its structural makeup continuously modifies the distribution of mineral salts. Chemical reserves of bones produce a renewal of calcium and phosphorus. Contrary to cartilage, tiny arteries irrigate the bones.

The skeletal structure is also subject to the influence of male hormones. The maturation of the skeleton during adolescence testifies to their fundamental impact. It is well established that a defect of male hormones induces a slenderness ratio of the bones and that excellent hormonal secretion gives a robust skeletal constitution.

When growing old, the bone structure weakens for four essential reasons caused by a lack of male hormones:

• Bone vascularization consists of a network of thin arteries reaching osseous ends. They take part in the generalized arteriosclerosis. The consequence is poor oxygenation of the articulations.

• Skeletal structures break up gradually. The collagenous fibers and the fundamental substance* take part in the degradation that strikes all protein structures of the organism.

• Calcium is badly fixed on support tissue, causing the bone porosity.

• Rarefaction of bone tissue is called *osteoporosis*. The bone is the seat of permanent remodeling. Its integrity depends on the balance between destruction and construction in the skeletal substance. Cortisol secreted by the suprarenal glands accentuates the process of decay. The structure of the skeleton depends on testosterone. At the time of menopause, the effects of cortisol exceed the constructive properties of testosterone, and osteoporosis develops.

In women, the osseous loss is accentuated with age and the lack of testosterone. There is a linear relationship between the plasma testosterone level and bone density.

The diagnosis of osseous brittleness is obtained by radiographs, which invariably show transparency of the bones, evidence of their brittleness. To see the decalcification of bones with X-rays, one needs a calcium deficit of approximately 30 percent. Thus, the radiological diagnosis is too late. Today, a more precise method of examination of bone density is available, quantitative computed tomography, which makes early diagnosis of osteoporosis possible and facilitates tracking of the regression of this degenerative phenomenon with the treatment of male hormones.

Years of rheumatism and joint pain precede the osteoporosis. With time, bone tissue is packed, and a woman with androgenic menopausal

---

* The collagenous fibers and the fundamental substance consist of proteins (see chapter 17).

disease sometimes loses several centimeters in height. Her bones become fragile, like glass. The least fall results in fractures.

The teeth are implanted in bone and fixed by ligaments. These structures degenerate, as does the structure of the body when testosterone is lacking. Tooth loosening is worsened by a lack of dental hygiene and excessive absorption of sugars, leading to the detachment of the gums and the formation of purulent pockets around dental roots.

Hormonal influences on connective tissue in the changes of aging have been known since 1958 [1].

In a 2011 cardiovascular health study, researchers from the Division of Endocrinology, University of Pennsylvania School of Medicine, Philadelphia, Pennsylvania, noted that a higher serum free testosterone concentration in older women was associated with greater bone mineral density and lean body mass and a decreased weight of total fat [2].

The harmful effects of estrogens in menopausal women have been known since 2002 [3]. In 2015, doctors who were concerned about the damage caused by treatment with estrogen or progesterone began prescribing bisphosphonates, which have some effect on strengthening the bone structure. However, these treatments are not always effective [4].

The lack of male hormones is a cause of osseous brittleness in women.

19

Skin Wrinkles

The skin plays a significant role in the organism. In the adult man, its weight can vary between thirteen and twenty-two pounds for a surface of 1.6 square meters. The skin has the advantage of being able to be observed in depth without difficulty, and the modifications caused by age are visible as soon as they appear after age forty-five years.

The cutaneous coating is a structure containing different elements. The epidermis is the outer of the two layers that make up the skin, the inner layer being the dermis.

The epidermis consists of superimposed cell layers; the deepest are flexible, and the superficial cells constitute the cornified layer—these separate from the deep layer as a result of burning (sunburn), forming blisters. In a healthy state, cornified cells flake off as a powder.

The major part of the skin, the dermis, contains many elastic fibers that are cutaneous tensioners responsible for smooth skin. Deep cells of the dermis produce a grease that constitutes a protective coating against the cold.

The skin contains two significant types of glands, ones that secrete greases (sebaceous glands) and others that secrete sweat (sudoriferous glands).

The sebaceous glands are in the deep part of the skin and are generally attached to hairs. Relatively rare on the chest, the neck, and the palms and soles, they are, on the contrary, numerous in certain areas, such as the scalp and the nose; there, one finds four hundred glands or more per square centimeter of human skin.

The sudoriferous glands are small tubes, inserted in the deep part of the skin, that cross the skin surface. There are approximately two hundred sudoriferous glands per square centimeter of skin, and their full number is three million for the whole of the cutaneous coating. The system of sudoriferous organs secretes about one liter of sweat per day; it can provide five to six liters or more.

The skin protects the organism from shocks and chemical aggression. It plays a significant role in thermal regulation, breathing, and elimination of the waste (e.g., urea, rock salts) of the organism. Extremely rich in nervous terminations, the skin is an organ of sensitivity and reflectivity.

The skin and its annexes are large consumers of male hormones. Old skin is characteristic of a woman with androgenic menopausal disease. Degenerative demonstrations are multiple. They are seen by the naked eye and draw attention, but it is possible to mitigate the effects with suitable hormonal treatment. With age, the superficial part of the skin thins. There are atrophied zones and young skin. With advanced age, the skin becomes extremely fine particularly on the back of the hands and the legs. In old age, the skin reduces to the thickness of a cigarette paper. It is also poorly irrigated, bloodless, and pale.

Young skin is elastic; old skin is not. Cutaneous elasticity is a result of the quality of collagenous fibers, elastic fibers, and dermal muscles.* With age, the collagenous tissues become rigid, and elastic fibers lose their elasticity. The phenomenon usually begins around age forty-five years but can occur from age thirty-five.

---

* The dermal muscles are superficial and are inserted in the deep part of the skin.

With time, the skin of the thorax tends to begin slipping, the inner side of the arms floats when one raises them horizontally, and the inner part of the thighs floats like a flag.

The dermal muscles take part in the generalized muscular atrophy of *androgenic menopausal disease.* There are muscles in the eyelids, the lips, the cheeks, the face, and the neck. All the muscles of mimicry are atrophied gradually by a lack of male hormones. The folded skin tends to hang. Drooping upper eyelids produce slanting eyes.

The drooping lower lip gives projects the image of a sulky person. The upper lip narrows and presents many vertical wrinkles.

Drooping cheeks result in jowls along the jaw. The face has vertical creases above the root of the nose and a succession of horizontal lines. The neck is folded. The lifelessness of the dermal muscles accentuates expression wrinkles, which become increasingly deeper because of muscular weakness. This reality can be masked when the face is invaded by fat, appearing as joviality (one may fear that losing weight will cause wrinkles to appear). The look of an untreated woman is marked by a kind of unhappiness or false airs.

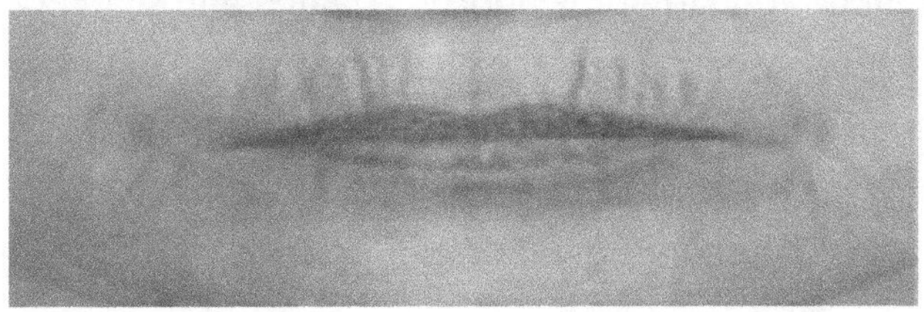

Fig. 24

Lip wrinkles.

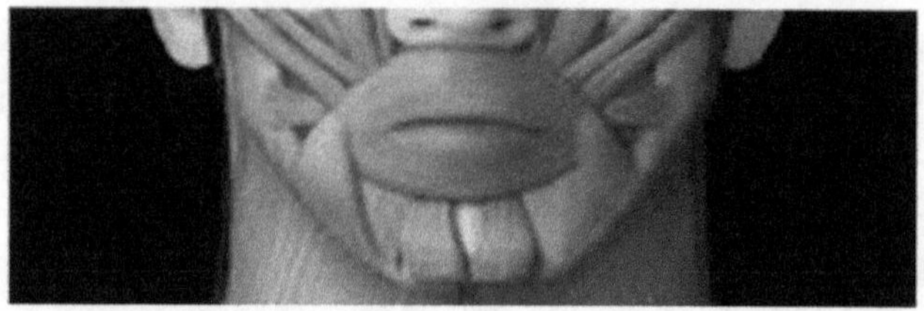

Fig. 25

Normal lip musculature.

Injection of a collagenous substance in wrinkles is popular today. The result is only temporary. Treatment with mesterolone maintains the elastic qualities of the skin and the lip muscles; it constitutes a real, permanent biochemical muscular facelift.

The production of sweat drops spectacularly after approximately age sixty. The water provision of the skin is compromised and drying of the skin is always present. This causes an incapacity to sweat and, consequently, intolerance to heat, accompanied by a fine exfoliative powder made up of dead cells. There is a reduction in the secretion of sebum by* the sebaceous glands [1].

Skin that renews too slowly is poorly irrigated and scarcely defended against infection. Most common is the consequence of colonization by a fungal organism, *Candida albicans*. It develops between the toes, within the circumference of the nails in the feet and fingers, and the cutaneous folds. Itching and burning follow, requiring antifungal treatment.

The skin contains specialized cells (melanocytes) charged with making the pigment melanin, which is responsible for tanning of the

* Sebum is a fat, is smooth, and contains protein substances; it is a product of secretion of the sebaceous glands and the waste of secreting cells.

skin. The melanin protects the skin from solar rays. The skin browns more, especially when the activity of the melanocytes is high. Aging of the skin appears with excessive and localized accumulations of melanin pigment. Brown spots make their appearance on the back of the hands, the forearms, the face, and the scalp. They are of variable size and form. They are commonly called "flowers of the cemetery."

In a woman with androgenic menopausal disease, the skin manufactures less and less melanin pigment; it reddens but does not brown, making exposure to the sun unbearable.

The skin of older women is also prone to small, spontaneous bleedings caused by the relaxation of cutaneous support tissue. The protection of the small, fragile dermal vessels not being assured, their walls tear with the least stretching or the least trauma. Healing of these lesions causes star-shaped white scars.

Hair and nails constitute the annexes of the skin. Hairs renew after a long time. Although the eyelashes and eyelids have only one short life, the hairs can persist from three to five years. New hairs replace them after their loss. Hair grows from 0.2 to 0.4 millimeters per day. On the leg, hairs lengthen 1.5 millimeters per week, those of the pubis and the armpits, 2.2 millimeters.

With age, hair tends to become sparse on the arms, legs, chest, armpits, and pubis because its growth depends on male hormones. Hair bleaches from a lack of melanin pigment. Hair growth relies on the activity of the thyroid gland, whose insufficiency can be suspected when hair loss is abnormal.

Nails are corneous plates that protect the ends of the fingers and toes. They consist of a protein, keratin. Usually, the nails must are hard. Their growth is practically indefinite. In women, growth is more active between five and thirty years of age. Growth is from approximately 1 millimeter per week for the fingernails and 0.25 millimeters for toenails. When male hormones are lacking, the nails become thin, cracked, and breakable. They do not grow anymore and are the site of fungal infections.

20

Shortness of Breath

With age, it is not so easy to extinguish all the candles on the birthday cake by blowing only once, especially when they are numerous. The test is familiar, and one is delighted when their grandmother succeeds after several times because it is, for her, a sign of great vitality.

The gaseous exchange between blood and the air depends primarily on the lung, which resembles a considerable sponge full of air. The cavities of this sponge consist of cells with small walls. Capillaries irrigate each cell, whose walls are thin.*

The cells are supported by tiny conjunctive tissues that ensure a certain elasticity of the lung. Inhalation depends on the respiratory muscles, which cause the expansion of the lungs. During exhalation, which is a passive phenomenon, the lung returns in on itself as a result of the elastic formations that surround the cells. The maximum quantity of air expelled after a maximum inhalation is 3.8 liters.

Chronic pulmonary emphysema is a permanent dilation of the air cells and the small bronchi. The capacity of lung ventilation is reduced, leading to poor air renewal. The thorax takes the shape of a barrel, and the neck seems too short. The respiratory movements are limited or even absent. One with emphysema cannot manage to extinguish a match. The breath is missing. Speaking is also challenging. The

---

* The entire surface of the alveolar walls is estimated at ninety square meters in men, and the maximum surface of the opened capillary network is 140 square meters. The gaseous exchange is made only by the diffusion between the air and the content of gas in the blood.

oxygen–blood transfer surface is reduced, creating extra work for the heart.

The principal mechanism of emphysema caused by aging is a loss of elasticity of the lung's conjunctive structure. During exhalation, the lung can no longer manage to retract entirely. The generalized aging of conjunctive tissue acts at the pulmonary level. See the discussion of the mechanism of this degeneration in chapter 17.

Senile emphysema is worsened by tobacco use, which provokes complex chemical reactions, also leading to the destruction of pulmonary elastic tissue.

The traditional treatment of emphysema is the drainage of the bronchi, bronchodilator drugs, antibiotics, and respiratory rehabilitation. As always, this treatment bearing on the consequences of emphysema, not the cause.

By acting on the elastic tissue of the lungs, male hormones can prevent chronic emphysema and the shortness of breath caused by age. The result will be more effective if treatment begins at the appearance of the first symptoms.

21

Metamorphoses of the Silhouette

Abdominal Bloating

The woman with androgenic menopausal disease tends to “inflate,” and her silhouette changes (see the figure 19, page 108).

The volume of the abdomen overloaded with fat increases further because of gases accumulated in high quantity in the digestive tract. Distension is capricious. In the beginning, it appears temporarily. The buttocks inflate first, then, with years, the belly. In men, the abdomen swells first, then, with years, the buttocks. In short, menopausal women look like men with *androgenic disease of andropause*. The stomach remains distended.

Gradually, the distension reproduces each day and intensifies during the day. In the evening, swelling is at its height, and then it disappears during the night. Lastly, the belly remains distended permanently, almost simulating pregnancy. A telling characteristic is that this kind of distension does not reabsorb after the elimination of gas and stools.

Digested food and the accompanying gases must cross eight meters of the intestine, on average, before being evacuated by the contraction of an important musculature.[*] With aging, the intestinal muscles

---

[***] The motor system of the digestive tract consists of the musculature of the small and large intestines. The small intestine measures approximately 6.5 meters and comprises fifteen to sixteen intestinal handles. It is made of a surface layer with longitudinal muscle fibers and a deep layer with circular fibers.
The length of the large intestine is 1.5 meters, on average. Like the small intestine, it is composed of two muscular layers.

degenerate in a woman, just like the whole of her musculature (chapter 11). This is the result of an insufficiency of male hormone secretion. It follows the atonality of the intestinal muscle fibers, which become unable to contract normally. Consequently, distension becomes permanent.

Traditional treatment of gas excess in the belly uses drugs that have the property to fix gases. Coal of vegetable origin is still used for this purpose. Once more, this treats the gas excess, a consequence of the distension, not the *atonic intestinal musculature*, the cause of distension. It is common to see the waist measurement of a swollen woman decrease in a few weeks thanks to treatment with mesterolone, while the possible weight loss previously did not yet influence the roundness.

Mesterolone stimulates the bowel muscles of a woman with menopausal disease and prevents the distension.

22

Kidney Failure

The kidneys are filtering stations that purify the blood of the toxic wastes of metabolism. Urea is the principal waste produced from protein degradation. Degeneration provoked by androgenic menopausal disease induces two mechanisms that involve the progressive destruction of the kidneys. Initially, arteriosclerosis of the renal arteries, followed by hypertension in the renal cavities. These two pathologies lead to renal insufficiency and possibly death by uremia.

The renal arteries take part in the degenerative process, which spreads gradually throughout the whole of the arterial network (chapter 12). This results in a lack of oxygen in renal tissue, which atrophies, causing a small, sclerotic kidney. Renal sclerosis, in turn, leads to two phenomena that are extremely damaging for the organism, one from excess, the other by default of secretion of the renal tissue.

Kidney degeneration results in the release of an enzyme,* renin, that causes an increase in the production of hypertensive hormones, thus worsening hypertension and arteriosclerosis.

Also, the sick kidney becomes unable to secrete a necessary hormone, erythropoietin, that stimulates the formation of red blood cells. This phenomenon causes and worsens anemia in women with androgenic menopausal disease.

---

* The enzyme is a protein substance that facilitates and increases a biochemical reaction.

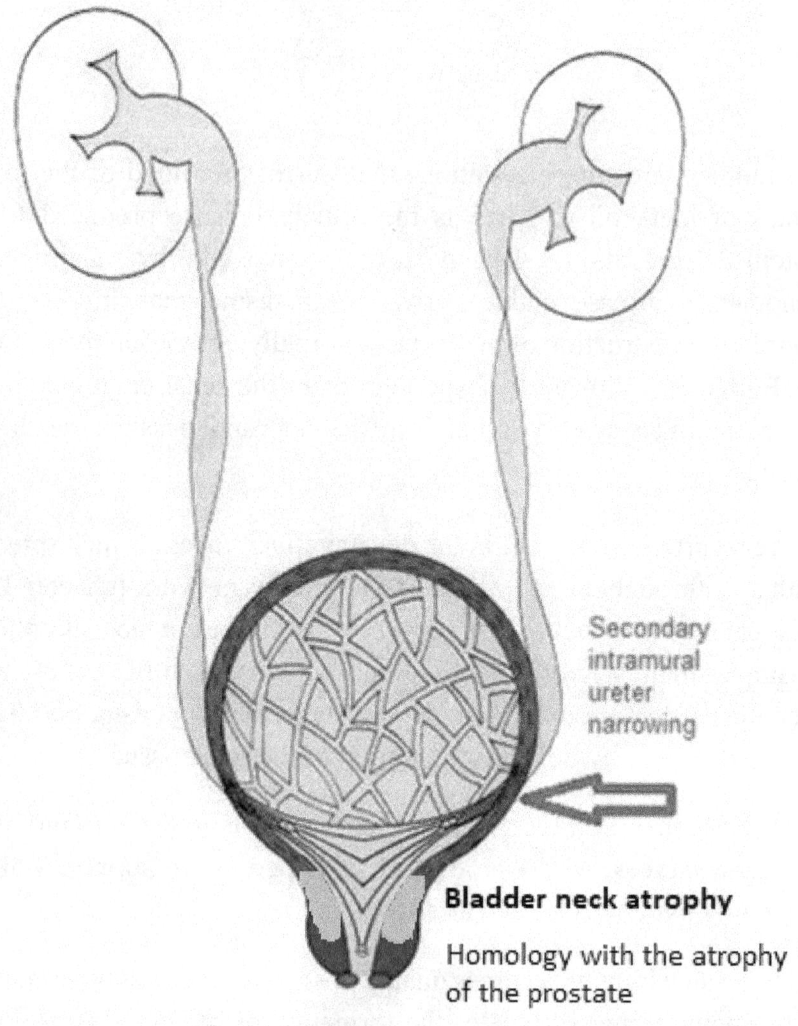

Fig 26

Atrophy and sclerosis of the bladder neck constitute an obstacle for urination. The vesical muscle reacts and hypertrophies. The

ureterotrigonal musculature also thickens. The diameter of the intravesical ureter narrows, and ureters dilate upstream.
By crossing the renal filter, blood eliminates the excess of water and waste of the organism to produce urine, which flows in the renal cavities before being propelled by the ureters into the bladder. From there, it is emitted outwardly by the urethra.
The urinary tract is a set of flexible systems. Bladder neck fibrosis is a permanent obstacle to urination. Fibrosis destroys not only the bladder but also the elements above it: the ureters, renal cavities, and kidneys.

The bladder reacts to a bladder neck obstacle by hypertrophying its musculature initially, and it becomes completely flaccid when the obstruction persists with time.

This pathology provokes another, lesser-known one, the deformation of the ureteral valve (ureterotrigonal valve), whose primary role is to prevent the backward flow of urine toward the kidney. This valve tightens initially; with time, it dislocates. The curious reader will find an explanation I did fifty years ago, and which is easy to assimilate [1].

The deformation of the ureteral valve constitutes an obstacle to urine flow toward the bladder. This phenomenon causes hypertension in the renal cavities, with a series of subsequent specific disorders.

Renal colic, generally due to a ureter obstruction by a calculus, is very painful. When there is a bladder neck obstacle, the musculature of the ureter contracts at its terminal segment in the bladder, causing renal colic in the absence of the calculus.* This phenomenon, little known,

* Colic is a pain that is felt in the internal organs of the belly.

explains certain renal colic cases whose cause is not evident. It is necessary to consider it in cases of repeating renal colic and in cases of bilateral renal colic.

The ideal urea level in the blood is from twenty-five to thirty milligrams per hundred milliliters of plasma. When the urinary tract is blocked, even partially, pressure increases in the renal cavities, impairing filtration and purification. A certain quantity of urea turns over in the general circulation, increasing its concentration in the blood. This explains the progressive rise in the urea level.

Renal degradation progresses gradually, even if the bladder neck obstruction is not continuous, because the urinary tract's flexible system distends, compromising the propulsion of urine. In the normal state, the urinary tract must always be free. An obstacle to the flow of urine, apparently undeveloped, constitutes an abnormal resistance that provokes, with time, the destruction of the kidneys. This concept is not always understood. It is, however, essential because obstruction of the urinary tract, even moderate, is incompatible with a long life.

It is necessary to be wary of urea levels that oscillate permanently around forty milligrams per hundred milliliters of plasma. When the urea level reaches this higher limit, a complete urological checkup is necessary.

If bladder neck obstruction remains, the urine that cannot be evacuated mixes with blood, and a high concentration causes uremia. The term *uremia* refers to a bankruptcy of the excretory function of the kidney, and the blood urea rises above fifty milligrams per hundred milliliters of plasma.

Death by uremia is relatively peaceful. The patient falls asleep, urea having gradual properties like sleeping pills. It is by making this observation that the idea came to manufacture barbiturates* from urea. The soothing properties of urea explain tiredness and disorders of memory and creativity when its level starts to rise in the blood. These symptoms constitute a real alarm bell.

Despite a standard health evaluation, migraines and giddiness, with or without accompanying tiredness, must make one think of hypertension in the renal cavities, a generally ignored and, consequently, unresearched pathology.

Ureters and renal cavities under excessive tension cause turbid reflexes of intestinal contraction. Bad digestion and distension of the belly are very frequent. One needs this knowledge to avoid taking unnecessary digestive powders over the years. The blocked urinary tract causes retention of water. It can reach several liters and cause leg edema. Conservation of water of two or three liters is already significant. It appears at the places where the skin is thinnest. The swelling of the eyelids must draw attention.

A simple blood test makes the diagnosis of renal insufficiency. One can then take an X-ray of the urinary tract (intravenous urography) to check its state after injecting an iodized solution into the arm. A few minutes later, it penetrates the urinary tract, which is visualized and shows the characteristic anomalies.

Bladder neck obstacles and sclerosis of the renal arteries cause progressive renal failure in women with menopausal disease.

---

* A barbiturate is an acid whose derivatives are used as sedatives (e.g., Veronal, Gardenal).

23

Hearing Loss and Vision Troubles

The sound that strikes the tympanum is transmitted in the ear by a chain of small bones articulated between them. Deprived of male hormones, they degenerate like the whole of bone tissue. The weakening of hearing announces impending deafness.

Vision Troubles

The most frequent vision pathologies are as follows:

- Presbyopia
- Cataract
- Glaucoma
- Retinal detachment
- Age-related macular degeneration (AMD)

Eye troubles in women with menopausal disease are the result of severe vascular modifications (chapter 12), sclerosis phenomena (chapter 17), glucose disturbances (chapter 8), and calcium disturbances as consequences of the insufficient secretion of male hormones.

The adaptation of vision depends, consequently, on a whole system of muscles whose tonicity is necessary for correct vision. The generalized involution of the muscles at the time of menopause does not spare ocular tissues. Eye troubles that appear at around age forty-five sound the alarm for the hormonal decline.

If one knows the importance of the influence of male hormones on the arterial network, can one neglect preventive hormonal treatment? Eye troubles in women with androgenic menopausal disease are the result of critical vascular modifications, sclerosis phenomena, and glucose and calcium disturbances. They are the consequences of insufficient secretion of male hormones.

In 1998, I advised a seventy-year-old woman, who had experienced hemorrhagic losses caused by an "unnecessary hormone replacement therapy" (HRT), to check her male hormones. Unfortunately, she followed her attending physician's advice to do nothing. Later, within years, she developed retinal detachment and is now almost blind.

HRT and Hearing Loss

Hearing problems are common among older people, and centers for hearing studies are increasing as the population ages.

Extensive research demonstrated that women who receive HRT lose more hearing than untreated women. Thus, they must escape from monolithic medical habits with the use of traditional HRT.

Hearing results from the action of a whole series of muscles activating a series of ossicles. The lack of testosterone causes widespread muscle atrophy, and the muscles of the ear do not escape this degeneration. It is the same for the ear's ossicles, which are altered by a lack of testosterone.

In 2017, Curhan and colleagues from the Channing Division of Network Medicine, Department of Medicine, Brigham and Women's Hospital, Harvard Medical School, Boston, Massachusetts, demonstrated that among postmenopausal women, oral HRT was associated with a higher risk of hearing loss. A longer duration of use was associated with a higher risk [1].

24

Immune Deficiency, AIDS, and Cancer

The media frequently announce accidents causing hip fractures in famous older women by specifying that it will take them many months of readjustment after hip replacement surgery. One or two years later, the media announce the death of the same famous older women following a lung infection. The chronology from hip fracture to death caused by a lung infection is common.

Testosterone stimulates immunity. The reduction in androgens induces a decrease in the production of lymphocytes, thus supporting the appearance of infection and cancer [1–3].

Testosterone is a controller of immunity, a property that allows the body to resist some disease-causing agents.

AIDS

Androgens can be more critical in patients who have AIDS, especially when they are weak, experience pain with physical effort, and have low lymphocyte levels.

This protective action of androgens on the globules was shown in 1997 by S. A. Klein and his collaborators. A thirty-seven-year-old man was in an extreme state of leanness. After three weeks' treatment with an androgen (1 alpha-dihydrotestosterone), the destruction of lymphocytes was reduced by 34 percent compared to the beginning of the therapy. At the same time, his general and nutritional condition was remarkably improved [4].

In 2009, a publication of the Program on Developmental Endocrinology and Genetics of the National Institutes of Health in Bethesda, Maryland, showed the prolongation of lymphocytes' telomeres under the influence of androgens [5]. Telomeres protect chromosomes from damage, and a shorter leukocyte telomere length is a marker of advancing biological age. Telomerase is involved in the size of telomeres. New studies about hormonal links with telomerase and stem cells are now necessary for older women.

Cancer

According to the World Health Organization, cancer is a significant cause of death in the world, causing 9,555,027 million deaths in 2018.

One area of immunity research concerns the prevention and treatment of tumors. Today, considerable progress has been made in the comprehension of cancer's mechanisms, thanks to the work of James Allison and Tasuku Honjo. They received the Nobel Prize in Physiology or Medicine in 2018 for their discovery of cancer treatment by inhibiting negative immune regulation. Immunotherapy is regarded, more and more, as an alternative therapy. Specific tumors are even able to be cured by treatments using the tools of immunity, and the pharmaceutical industry has already put on the market anticancer drugs that have been approved by the US Food and Drug Administration (FDA).

The prevention of tumors can benefit from preventive treatment with melatonin, according to the work of Russel J. Reiter of the University of Texas Health Science Center at San Antonio [6].

Without prevention, the future of older people is either to degenerate due to arteriosclerosis and Alzheimer's disease or to develop tumors.

We have already seen that arteriosclerosis can be prevented. Its preventive treatment with mesterolone as early as the age of forty is decisive. This result will be all the more impressive by preventing the development of tumors if melatonin is taken at the same time as mesterolone [7].

25

Depression

A woman with androgenic menopausal disease sees a complete upheaval of her mental structures because the brain, a large consumer of male hormones, is not stimulated and degenerates. Depression settles in and causes the appearance of many negative symptoms that will affect daily life. The World Health Organization estimates that experiences of depression affect more than 350,000,000 individuals each year [1]. Fifty percent of doctor visits are a result of this disease, whose cause is, curiously, not known. The action of male hormones on the nervous system should make reflect us on that.

Today, we see the importance of male hormones for nerve cells and behavior. A whole work would be necessary to develop the subject; studies are numerous and exceed the framework of this book. But the sections that follow will reveal an unexpected aspect of sex hormones, which control not only our sexuality but also our thoughts, our moods, and our behaviors.

Studies have shown the impressive concentration of sex hormones in the nervous system. The demonstration was made in rats by injections of dihydrotestosterone marked with radioactive isotopes. Histological cuts showed localization of the labeled molecules in various nervous structures of sacrificed animals. Brain cells, the cerebellum, the spinal cord, and cranial nerve cells contain potent male hormone molecules. Male hormones are concentrated primarily in the motor cells that control action and movement. Female hormones are mainly present in sensitive nerve cells.

Male hormones are also present in the other components of the brain, for example, in the arteries and ventricles.*

The presence of male hormones in the brain is so vital that one can question their role in nervous system degenerative diseases when they are insufficient.

There are also cerebral centers of sexuality. Their sensitivity to the action of male and female sex hormones explains the differences in sexual behaviors. Behavior depends, consequently, on the effect of sex hormones on the nerve cells.

Much of the male's body systems also depend on testicular secretion. Researchers studied the testosterone level in thirty-six prisoners divided into three groups [2]. The first group consisted of men having shown a chronic aggressiveness: violent physical aggression, attacks, crimes, and still uttering aggressive words and threats despite their imprisonment. The second group was composed of socially dominant men occupying a raised situation in the social hierarchy, white-collar criminals imprisoned for robbery, drugs, or illicit money—lastly, the third group comprised of nonviolent prisoners who were socially non-dominant.

The experiment showed that the most aggressive men had the highest testosterone levels, and the least aggressive men had the lowest levels. The socially dominant men had an average hormonal level. The hormone levels were characteristic of each individual and varied little over the days of the study. The most aggressive men were particularly insensitive to anxiety [2].

---

* The ventricles are cerebral cavities that contain cerebrospinal fluid.

All mental faculties diminish gradually when male hormones are lacking. Creativity decreases first in artists, painters, sculptors, writers, and so forth, then disappears at the time of androgenic menopausal disease. Hormonal treatment restarts their faculties of creation, making their works more durable and more beautiful.

In a normal woman, the capacity for fixing memory varies according to age. A three-year-old child remembers a series of three numbers. At four years, the child retains four. Toward six to eight years, the child memorizes five numbers; at ten years, six numbers, and at fourteen years, a series of seven figures. The series that a healthy adult can remember hovers around seven digits.

Traditional treatment of depression uses antidepressant drugs. Among them, inhibitors of monoamine oxidase, a cerebral enzyme, are commonly prescribed. They are not always well supported, however, because they can cause giddiness, headaches, nausea, and constipation. It is interesting to point out that *testosterone is a natural inhibitor of monoamine oxidase*. The disappearance of the depressive symptoms can be obtained in a few days as soon as the brain contains male hormones [3].

Memory loss is one of the primary symptoms of androgenic menopausal disease. Curiously, recent facts are forgotten initially, whereas images of the past remain in memory. A woman with androgenic menopausal disease forgets instantaneously the answer that she received to the question she repeats, without realizing it, sometimes on several occasions. Under these conditions, it can become complicated to continue in one's occupation. Women with androgenic menopausal disease are unable to retain their ideas. A progressive loss of mental faculties can result in these women becoming unemployed, unable to reintegrate themselves into society.

In the morning, the woman with androgenic menopausal disease rises tired. During the day, she drags. At the limit, she is tired of being tired, with all her cerebral structures lacking male hormones. She becomes unable to use the whole of her intellectual faculties and does not perceive any goal to realize. "To act" and "to want" are lost concepts because the vital energy has disappeared. Instinctively, she knows that the countdown started and that there is nothing to hope for anymore. How often I've heard, "I am tired," "I quit the business," "My job is rotten, I do not know what to do," or, "I thought about running for election, but I gave up." I've heard the same women say, after hormonal treatment, "To give up my business? I do not think of it anymore. On the contrary, I created a new one," or, "I reconsidered my job; I am leaving for new horizons," or, "Finally, I ran and won the election." Those results are something completely refreshing.

There is no sexual instinct without male hormones. The absence of libido can occur suddenly; generally, though, it settles down gradually, and certain women accept it the older they get. Others seek to be reassured. They think that the phenomenon is momentary. Then they begin looking for all kinds of excuses. Little by little, concern appears. Sexual intercourse becomes increasingly rare; months pass without any sexual desire. The repercussions in the couple's relationship are inevitable, especially when the partner is younger. Comprehension quickly gives way to suspicions: "He misleads me," or, worse, "He does not like me anymore."

Consequently, the vicious circle of mutual incomprehension starts with, on the one hand, an increasingly ice-cold woman and, on the other side, a woman haunted by a fear of failure due to lack of desire. With time, the situation becomes intolerable, even dramatic, and inevitably leads to the separation of the lovers. All of that would have arranged itself if the lack of hormones did not worsen the situation.

A woman must unceasingly protect herself from external aggressions by mobilizing her hormonal balance, which is controlled by the brain. The mechanism is always the same in all the circumstances of life: loss of a loved one, unemployment, bankruptcy, surgical procedure, burns, and conflict without exit. All reactions of the body to aggression were brilliantly described and proven by Canadian physiologist Hans Selye under the name of *general adaptation syndrome*, which one generally calls the *effects of stress*.

Everything starts with an alarm reaction that mobilizes the hormones of the suprarenal glands (cortisol and adrenaline), which are the hormones of urgency. At the same time, the secretion of male hormones rises, increasing aggressiveness and providing the energy reserves necessary for combat or escape (by increasing the muscles' metabolism). Then, if stress is prolonged or reproduced at too high of a frequency, the secretion of male hormones falls, leading to depression, with the incapacity to react. Under these conditions, a woman with androgenic menopausal disease constitutes a prey to stress because she is unable to mobilize her male hormones in enough quantity.

Morbid unhappiness without apparent cause is a natural consequence of androgenic menopausal disease. There is a gross disproportion between the futility of the reason and the intensity of the sadness and gloomy mood. Discouragement, dislike, and pessimism are parts of daily life, which seems dull, gray, and stripped of direction. Concern leads to anxiety, possibly with fear of the surrounding world.

Melancholy of women with androgenic menopausal disease is always present if not subjacent with various disorders. Women complaining about sexual disorders due to age very often take antidepressant drugs, their sexual failures being attributed, wrongly, to mood disorders. It is not so much the depression that should be erased, but the putting of the organism under pressure, which is different. Male hormones have the particularity of stimulating cerebral and sexual functions simultaneously.

A depression also appears with disorders of self-awareness. The feeling of not being oneself, losing standing, or not belonging to humanity anymore inevitably leads to withdrawal, isolation, and the impression of living under a bell. Incapacity to communicate causes ruptures with the external world, which appears increasingly hostile. The situation becomes complicated because of people's incomprehension at home or work, especially when nothing explains the odd and silent behavior. Charges are concise: "And yet she has everything to be happy about"; "She is a shirker"; "She has something in mind." Consequently, depression worsens; black thoughts appear and sometimes lead to suicide. Unfairly accusing the weak always seemed unbearable to me, mainly because the accusations often come from beings who are only strong in front of weak ones.

I met Susan, a forty-nine-year-old doctor, during an anti-aging congress. She was desperate.

She told me that she felt depressed, unable to react. She did not like her work anymore. Everything was too much. To her misfortune, her sexual desire had disappeared, and her lover was ten years younger. At a simple glance, she was overweight by around ten pounds. I advised her to do a blood test to determine her testosterone and dihydrotestosterone levels. A month later, she phoned me to confirm her low levels of testosterone and dihydrotestosterone. I proposed a simple treatment: it would be necessary to lose ten pounds with an appropriate diet and to take five milligrams of mesterolone a day continuously.

Even as a doctor, Susan was skeptical; she believed that her depression was the cause of all her misfortune, but the treatment seemed rather simple to her, so she said she would do what was necessary.

I saw her one year later at the next anti-aging congress; Susan had lost ten pounds, her blood tests had improved, she had recovered her sexual desire, and she was radiant. Finally, she realized that her troubles and her depression were the consequence of biochemical deterioration caused by her insufficiency of male hormones. She understood, henceforth, that she would carefully supervise her food and her male hormones. This was only the beginning.

Women are more than twice as likely as males to be afflicted by mood disorders, not only in the United States but also worldwide. They are more likely to experience mood disturbances, anxiety, and depression during times of hormonal flux, such as puberty, menopause, and perimenopause, indicating a sensitivity to hormonal changes. In 2014, two scientific studies emphasized the role of testosterone in those hormonal changes [4,5].

Production of male hormones decreases gradually and continuously over the years, causing a weakened and depressed older woman. However, this lack of production can occur in a few months; it is different for each person.

Sometimes, a complete study of the daily secretion of androgen hormones is necessary to show an insufficient production of male hormones. This study determines the levels of hormonal precursors and androgen hormones. The study also covers the metabolites in urine over twenty-four hours.

In the 1990s, doctors thought that the intake of dehydroepiandrosterone (DHEA) could overcome depression. DHEA is a testosterone precursor available freely in drugstores in the United States. In 1990, a study was undertaken by the Department of Psychiatry of New York University School of Medicine in which a depressed woman was given a considerable quantity of DHEA.

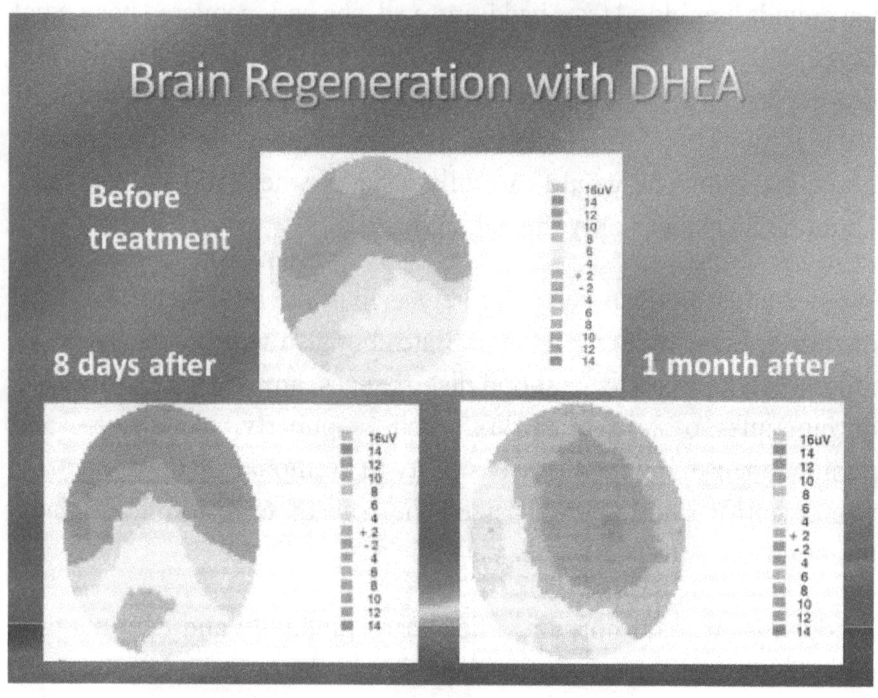

Fig. 27

Based on Bonnet and Brown [6].

The patient received 12.5 mg/kg/day (low dose) or 37 mg/kg/day (high dose) for two years. The patient weighed seventy kilos. With these incredibly high doses, DHEA converts into equally high doses of testosterone and dihydrotestosterone in the blood. This results in a rapid improvement of brain activity, as shown by the brain scan recordings before treatment, eight days after, and one month after (see the figure 27). Such doses of DHEA are inappropriate and dangerous. But it is remarkable to note the rapid improvement of brain activity. With the use of physiological doses of safe mesterolone in depressed women, their brain scans will also show this improvement. This study remains to be done and will be of the highest interest.

The problems with the use of DHEA are as follows:

- It is a chemical substance that is a precursor of hormones.
- It is transformed in the body into various substances with different purposes according to the administered doses (e.g., testosterone and estradiol, a female hormone) [7].
- It is not transformed directly into dihydrotestosterone (the potent sex hormone for men and women).
- It slows down the pituitary gland by producing contradictory hormonal substances according to the administered doses.
- It does not correspond to a well-defined pathology.
- It produces testosterone transformed into estradiol—a female hormone that is a proliferative hormone.
- It should not be sold without medical prescription.
- It is not the treatment for androgenic menopausal disease.

In 2018, Positron Emission Tomography (PET) was a non-invasive imaging tool used to evaluate the effects of hormonal therapy on specific downstream processes in the brain. [8].

26

Parkinson's Disease

A biochemical substance partly orders our movements. It is dopamine, secreted by specialized cells located in a center within the base of the brain (called the *substantia nigra or locus niger*). When destroyed, these cells do not secrete dopamine anymore; the musculature solidifies and is prone to shaking.

The Frozen Drug Addicts

William Langston, a neurologist at Santa Clara Valley Medical Center in Northern California, was stunned by the arrival to his office a motionless young man, as if frozen—mute, with large open eyes that did not blink.

One can understand the stupefaction of the other doctors consulted, who had never seen such a case before. By examining the girlfriend of the young man, Langston and his fellow neurologist, Phil Ballard, noted that she was in the same frozen state as him. They suspected a connection between the two cases.

By chance, Ballard went to a meeting arranged by one of his neurologist friends, James Tetrud, who told him that he, too, had seen two similar cases in his consultation.

The four "frozen" people were heroin addicts. Langston went on television to alert the community of the existence of illegal tainted heroin sold on the street. Following this, a spectator announced two other cases. Six individuals were "frozen."

Langston got samples of the remaining substance that the victims had injected. Analyses of the drug sold as heroin showed that it was a toxic synthetic product, MPTP,* which causes permanent symptoms of Parkinson's disease by destroying specific neurons in the black substance of the brain. Studies using this molecule are undertaken in monkeys.

The story of the frozen drug addicts was told with passion by William Langston and Jon Palfreman, a medical writer, in the book *The Case of the Frozen Addicts: How the Solution of an Extraordinary Medical Mystery Has Spawned a Revolution in the Understanding and Treatment of Parkinson's Disease* [1]. When a frozen addict dies, the autopsy shows the destruction of the cells secreting dopamine in the brain.

When the cells that secrete dopamine die or are damaged, one sees the appearance of motor disorders of progressive evolution. Parkinson's disease usually begins at age forty-five or fifty (ages for the beginning of the menopausal illness) or after. It is the second-most-frequent neurodegenerative disease after Alzheimer's disease.

Parkinson's disease provokes motor symptoms (e.g., shaking, muscular rigidity, slowness of movements) and nonmotor symptoms (e.g., constipation, disturbed sleep, emergencies to urinate, frigidity, dizzy spells, tiredness, depression, memory disorders). This disease results from the lack of production of dopamine by specialized cells localized in the depth of the brain. One of the causes of the destruction of the cells producing dopamine resides in the fact that they no longer receive blood because of arteriosclerosis (chapter 12).

---

* MPTP: 1-methyl, 4-phenyl, 1, 2, 3, 6-tetrahydro pyridine.

Testosterone could play a producing, determining role in biochemistry, even in the cells producing dopamine [2], or by improving blood circulation to these cells. An interesting area of research is the daily androgen production in women who have Parkinson's disease.

Also, treatment with androgens will decrease the tendency toward depression and will limit the need to take "antidepressants."

Normal Production of Androgens	Insufficient Production of Androgens
↓	↓
Tiny, permeable arteries	Tiny, blocked arteries
↓	↓
Normal cells secreting dopamine	Cells secreting dopamine destroyed
↓	↓
Normal production of dopamine	Insufficient production of dopamine
↓	↓
Normal movements	Shaking

Table 18

Facing the full extent of the disasters provoked by arterial rigidity, as outlined in the table 18, can one neglect its prevention with androgen hormones?

27

Dementias and Alzheimer's Disease

Alzheimer's Disease in Short

Dementias are the consequence of a progressive diminution of blood flow in the brain, producing atrophy and destruction of the brain tissue. Those phenomena provoke secondary lesions (senile plates), amyloid deposits, and immune reactions in Alzheimer's disease, which is a neurodegenerative pathology.

Alzheimer's disease is generally the consequence of poor irrigation of certain parts of the brain where memory concentrates: the amygdala and the hippocampus.

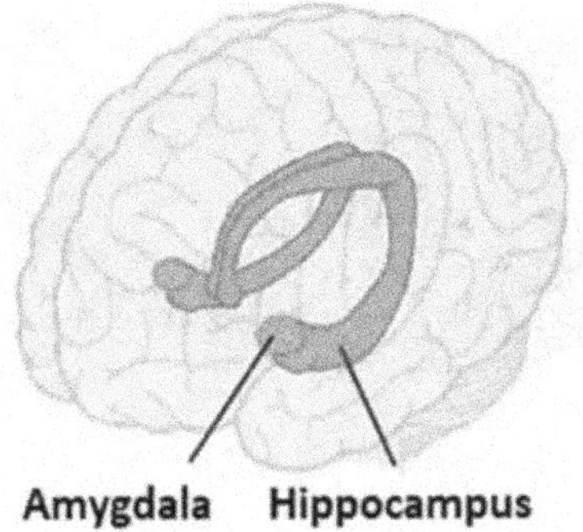

Fig. 28

Amygdala and hippocampus in the depths of the brain.

Arteriosclerosis is a disease of aging, producing a progressive narrowing of the brain arteries. This phenomenon starts around age

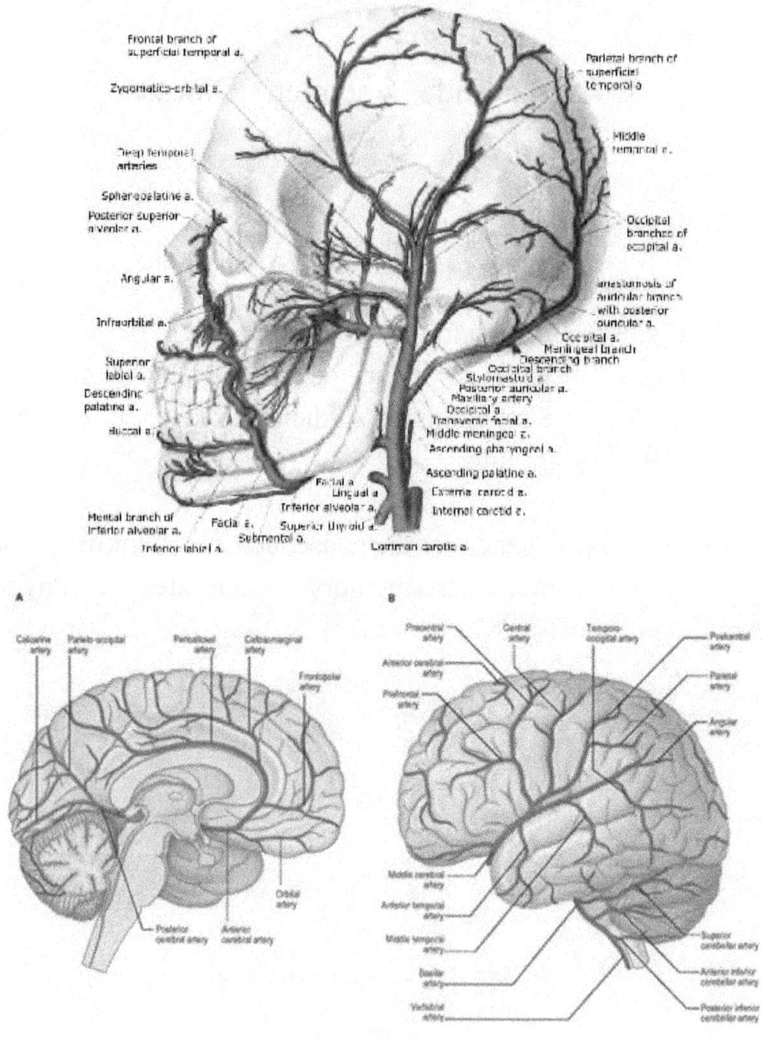

Fig. 29

Normal brain arteries.

When an arterial branch becomes clogged, the tissue of the irrigated area is destroyed.

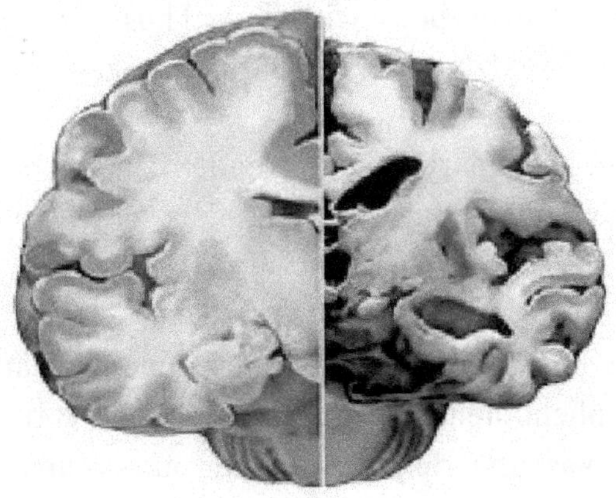

Fig. 30

Left: Healthy brain. Right: Alzheimer's brain tissue—the final stage.

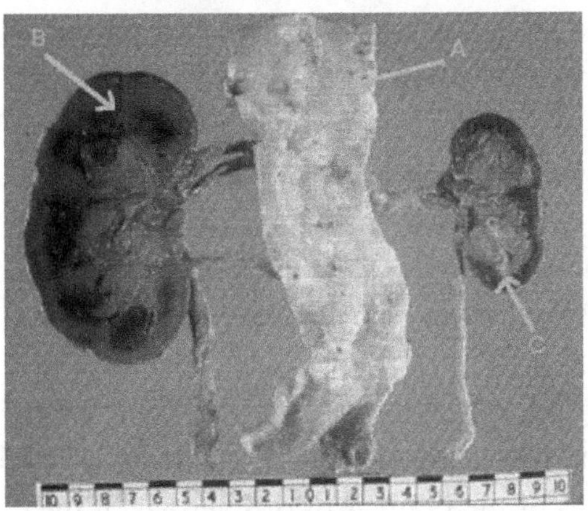

Fig. 31

Left (B): Healthy kidney. Right (C): Atrophied kidney following arterial stenosis and thus a progressive diminution of blood flow in the organ, producing atrophy and destruction of the kidney tissue.

forty and will reach everybody with time. Thus, the prevention of the pathology known as Alzheimer's disease must start around age forty.

The treatment of secondary lesions (senile plates), amyloid deposits, and immune reactions is hazardous and has mostly been abandoned [1].

Arteriosclerosis is a disease of aging, producing a narrowing of the arteries. This phenomenon starts around age forty and may be responsible for vascular disorders of various organs (hypertension, Parkinson's disease, vision and hearing troubles, etc.)

The progressive diminution of blood flow in the brain produces atrophy and destruction of the brain tissue.

Arteriosclerosis is a disease of aging that produces a progressive hardening and narrowing of the brain arteries. Over time, arteriosclerosis destroys the entire brain. The brain with Alzheimer's shown in the figure 30 is in the final stage.

As noted, the destruction of the brain starts around age forty and will reach everybody with time; thus, the prevention of dementia must start around age forty.

Arteriosclerosis, the cause of which is unknown, develops randomly in different areas of the brain. Arteriosclerosis of the cerebral arteries is a general phenomenon associated with dementia.

Depending on the location of the vascular involvement generally associated with dementia, the symptoms will be those of Alzheimer's disease, vascular dementia, or Parkinson's disease.

Different areas of the brain can be affected. In the beginning, destruction involves specific regions. For example, Alzheimer's disease is a form of dementia characterized by progressive memory loss over the years associated with secondary lesions (senile plates), amyloid deposits, and immune reactions. This pathology affects the amygdala and hippocampus in the depths of the brain.

For example, tremors characterize Parkinson's disease. This pathology affects the substantia nigra, which is a basal ganglia structure located in the midbrain.

Over time, arteriosclerosis destroys the entire brain.

How to Stop It?

Again, the destruction of the brain starts around age forty and will reach everybody with time; thus, the prevention of dementia must start around age forty.
A drug can only reach the diseased areas of the brain if the cerebral arteries are permeable. Research should start there.
Therefore, for natural molecules such as hormones or drug molecules to reach the brain cells, it is essential first to keep the cerebral arteries healthy, which is the right treatment t for the prevention of diseases of aging [2].

Alzheimer's Disease Facts and Figures

- Twenty years or more before symptoms appear, the brain changes of Alzheimer's may begin.
- In the United States, 5.8 million Americans are living with Alzheimer's dementia.

- Deaths from Alzheimer's increased by 145 percent between 2000 and 2017.
- The estimated cost of Alzheimer's and other dementias, including costs of health care, long-term care, and hospice, totaled $290 billion in 2019 [3].

Dementia Rates

The World Health Organization noted in 2019 that dementia affects about 50 million people worldwide, approximately 60 percent of whom live in low- and middle-income countries. They are about ten million new cases each year. Between 5 and 8 percent of the general population aged sixty or over has dementia at any given time.

The total number of people with dementia will reach 82 million in 2030 and 152 million in 2050. In low- and middle-income countries, the number of people with dementia will tend to continue to increase.

What Is Known

Contrary to popular opinion, brain degeneration is not the result of a continuous loss of nerve cells. The brain loses approximately ten thousand cells per day of the ten billion neurons* that constitute it. Consequently, the cellular loss represents only 3 percent of nervous cells over eighty years and does not seem to be responsible for the degeneration, with the remaining cells being sufficient enough. Degeneration is the consequence of the atrophy and disappearance of

---

* Neuron: nervous cell generally made up of a body of variable form and equipped with various prolongations, one of which, threadlike and longer than the others, is called the axon.

the ramifications that link the nervous cells, enabling them to communicate.

Male Hormones Regenerate Nerve Cells

In the 1970s and 1980s, researchers highlighted the brain's plasticity.

Philippe van den Bosch de Aguilar, a neurobiologist from the Catholic University of Leuven, Belgium, studied the brains of seven generations of rats over fifteen years, observing and counting the neurons. He noted that the brain's nerve cells develop new nervous terminations at around twenty-four months, a lifetime corresponding to eighty years in man. This study established a new concept: the older brain preserves the power of reactivity and plasticity.

Dick Swaab, from the Dutch Institute of Research on the Brain, showed the favorable influence of testosterone on rats' brains. Observation under the microscope indicated that nerve cells were well ramified in the young rat. These ramifications disappeared in the old rat but reappeared under the influence of testosterone, managed in the form of implants. The phenomenon is most probably the same in humans.

Nervous fibers are surrounded by a myelin[*] sheath that insulates them and protects them to support the propagation of nerve impulses, like plastic does around electric wires.

Today, it is possible to repair the nerve fibers damaged by the lack of myelin during degenerative diseases of the brain. In 2013, a group of researchers from different INSERM (the French National Institute of

---

[*] Myelin: substance made up of fats and proteins.

Health and Medical Research) units and various US universities described androgen receptors in the nerve cells of a mouse. These receptors constitute a therapeutic target for myelin repair of nerve brain cells, having lost this component of their structure when spontaneous myelin repair is no longer possible. This effect is probably due to the immune and anti-inflammatory, neuroprotective action of testosterone [4]. Consequently, it seems logical to me to analyze the androgen production in a woman presenting with degeneration of the nervous system, to be able to manage androgen treatment with full safety. Detection and hormonal treatment are necessary from the appearance of the primary symptoms to prevent definitive nerve damage.

Dementias

The World Health Organization (WHO) published the 2012 report "Dementia: A Public Health Priority," which mentions information about dementia [5]. Dementia is a syndrome that implies deterioration of memory, intellect, behavior, and the capacity to carry out activities of daily life. Worldwide, there are some 35.6 million people who have dementia. Each year, there are 7.7 million new cases. According to this WHO report, the number of people affected by dementia will triple in 2050, increasing the number of affected individuals to 115 million. Dementia is one of the leading causes of dependence in older adults in the world. Dementia has a physical, psychological, social, and economic impact on nursing staff, families, and society. Six percent of older people over age sixty-five are affected by a variable degree of dementia, caused by the deterioration of the nervous ramifications and the appearance of degenerative plates in the cerebral structures.

Variety of Dementias

There are four subtypes of dementia: Alzheimer's disease, vascular dementia, dementia with Lewy bodies, and frontotemporal dementia. The diagnosis must be interpreted with prudence because clear cases are rarer than mixed pathologies.

Alzheimer's Disease

Alzheimer's disease is the most common cause of dementia. It represents between 60 and 70 percent of the cases of dementia.

Generally Accepted Ideas

Despite a more thorough knowledge of Alzheimer's disease, many generally accepted ideas still circulate on this neurodegenerative pathology, among which are that Alzheimer's disease is a natural consequence of old age or that Alzheimer's disease is a quite specific and incurable degenerative disease. These assertions are vague and do not correspond to reality.

Various Forms of Alzheimer's Disease

The most common form is the nonhereditary or sporadic form. It accounts for 99 percent of cases. The other, very rare, form is the family or hereditary form.

Various Stages of Alzheimer's Disease

Alzheimer's disease passes through multiple phases, which will lead to death in eight to twelve years. The four stages are the light period, the moderate, the severe, and the final step.

Pathological Modifications in the Brain

Alzheimer's disease is characterized by the deposit of senile plates containing β-amyloid protein and by abnormal tangles of nervous ramifications in affected cerebral areas.

These anomalies cause immune reactions involving and aggravating cellular destruction [6–8].

Recent and Determining Scientific Discoveries

In 1999, researchers at Rockefeller University of New York and Cornell University of New York made an important discovery. They showed, using cultures of nerve cells, that testosterone reduces the secretion of the protein β-amyloid peptide [9].

This study concluded that androgens could protect against the development of Alzheimer's disease.

In 2001, the first clinical description of the increased levels of β-amyloid protein in the blood was published by a research team at the University of Western Australia in Perth [10]. They showed that chemical castration in men caused a drop in plasma estradiol and testosterone levels parallel to the rise in β-amyloid protein. The *Journal of the American Medical Association* published this capital discovery: "Chemical Andropause and Amyloid-Beta Peptide" (2001, 285: 2195–2196). This study shows that testosterone replacement can prevent or delay Alzheimer's disease.

In 2004, researchers at the University of Southern California studied the brain testosterone content in deceased men in two groups. The first group did not present neuropathology (group controls). The second group suffered from Alzheimer's disease or moderate neuropathology.

This study concluded that the cerebral tissue of patients who had Alzheimer's disease contained significantly less testosterone than the brains of men without a neurophysiological anomaly [11].

In 2008, Emily R. Rosario and Christian J. Pike of the Davis School of Gerontology of the University of Southern California, Los Angeles, published a review of scientific publications on Alzheimer's disease [12]. The conclusion of this review was as follows:

> Alzheimer's disease shows an abnormal accumulation of protein β-amyloid in the brain. Recent studies suggest the regulating action of androgens on the β-amyloid protein and development of Alzheimer's disease. Therapy with androgens may prevent and treat Alzheimer's disease.

In 2011, Emily Rosario and collaborators demonstrated decreased brain levels of androgen and estrogen hormones in men and women during healthy aging, which may be relevant to the development of Alzheimer's disease [13]. In the same year, an article in the *American Family Physician* noted the small effect of treatment with testosterone on Alzheimer's disease [14]. This conclusion is exact. Indeed, with destroyed nervous tissue, no effective drug exists. Male hormones are effective in the *prevention* of Alzheimer's disease before the destruction of nerve cells.

How to Direct the Treatment of Alzheimer's Disease with Androgens?

The clinical studies carried out to date are remarkable. They highlight the significant impact of testosterone on Alzheimer's disease [9–13]. There are, however, recent publications from eminent researchers who question the effectiveness of androgens in the treatment of

Alzheimer's disease [14]. The destruction of nerve cells is always definitive. How to solve these apparent contradictions?

The role of testosterone and androgens in treating and preventing Alzheimer's disease requires a more detailed approach. It seems useful to me to draw attention to the fact that the clinical studies only look at the testosterone level in the blood. That does not make it possible to have a precise idea of the levels of androgens. Future studies should evaluate daily androgen production. In men, a blood testosterone level of 600 ng/100 mL can correspond to a pathology. On the other hand, a level of 350 ng/100 mL can indicate nonpathological metabolism, not requiring a hormonal substitution.

The double-blind experimental setup is necessary for clinical studies. This makes it possible to have a general idea of the results while having eliminated the subjective factors. Such studies are convenient for direct research.

But I would like to draw attention to the hormonal singularity of each person who has Alzheimer's disease. It is advisable to make a detailed study of androgen metabolism **in each patient**. The singular study of androgens in each person presenting with Alzheimer's disease makes it possible to prescribe a precise and well-proportioned androgen treatment. Testosterone is not the only androgen available, and for women, mesterolone is the right drug. Administration of a standard testosterone dose is not conducive to treating each person. Standard doses always constitute a therapeutic approximation. The biology is singular for each patient and implies a peculiar treatment with androgens or a possible singular counterindication with this treatment. Failing this, a single and standard testosterone amount can lead to undesirable effects.

A better knowledge of therapy with androgens should be part of university education. The administered doses, in general, are often too weak or too strong. To consider a standard testosterone dose for each patient is not reasonable. The doses of insulin or thyroxin to treat diabetes or thyroid insufficiency are not the same across individuals. Future clinical studies and medication need a detailed analysis of androgen metabolism in people with Alzheimer's disease. This will probably make it possible to have a better understanding of the treatment and hormonal prevention of this disease.

The regularization of androgen metabolism is necessary from the appearance of the first symptoms of Alzheimer's disease. Upstream, the arrival of the early signs of the menopausal disease gives a signal. In 2012, researchers at the University of Tokyo and Hamamatsu University School of Medicine in Shizuoka, Japan, showed the beneficial effect of testosterone on cognitive function in mice and the inhibition of senescence of the vascular endothelial cells of the hippocampus* [15].

Destruction of nerve cells begins in the depths of the brain in the structure called the *hippocampus*. Then the destroyed cerebral tissue extends gradually into increasingly broad cerebral zones. Damage of the whole brain then causes inevitable death after many years of confusion and dementia.

For fifteen years, testosterone has already shown its neuroprotective effect on neuronal death, according to several scientific observations (see the previous discussion).

---

*Hippocampus: small cerebral convolution whose form represents the shape of a small fish of the same name. This structure is in the depths of the human brain. It is responsible for memory and space orientation. Nervous The nerve cells of the hippocampus can multiply during the adult life.

Mechanisms of Cerebral Lesions When the Production of Male Hormones Is Insufficient	
Normal Production of Androgens	Insufficient Production of Androgens
↓	↓
Tiny permeable arteries	Tiny blocked arteries
↓	↓
Normal nerve cells Active hormonal receivers	Destroyed nerve cells Destroyed hormonal receivers
↓	↓
Normal production of myelin New ramifications of nerve fibers	Abnormal production of myelin ↓ Ruptures of nerve fibers' ramifications ↓ Accumulation of β-amyloid proteins ↓ Autoimmunity reactions
Vascularization is standard in the whole brain. Receptors of androgens are activated generally in the whole brain.	In the beginning, vascularization is defective in the profound parts of the brain and then in its totality. Receptors of androgens are no longer activated in cerebral territories, flooded or not.
↓ Normal brain	↓ Dementias

In 2014, Chinese researchers studied the mechanism of the toxicity of β-amyloid protein on synaptic transmission* and the simultaneous effect of testosterone. Their discovery is of high importance. Researchers studied the hippocampus neuronal cells of rats in culture, set in contact with β-amyloid proteins and testosterone.

The general effect of β-amyloid protein† was that it lowered the effectiveness of the synaptic transmission.

The Chinese study confirmed the protective effect of testosterone on synaptic transmission in the presence of β-amyloid protein. Researchers made these discoveries in various institutions in the Republic of China [16].

The doctor confronted with Alzheimer's disease has very few means of treatment because the destruction of nerve cells is always definitive. Treatment of Alzheimer's disease is initially preventive. It is necessary to act from the beginning of the disease, such as when one forgets unceasingly where the keys are. Therapy with androgens at the beginning of Alzheimer's disease would represent significant progress because the condition would likely stop advancing at this stage. That would make it possible not to lose the keys all the time after age forty and avoid developing insanity after that. This approach would also make it possible to prevent many of the diseases of aging described in this book. Not counting the fundamental impact of testosterone on the maintenance of cerebral artery patency, can one neglect the regenerating effect of male hormones on the ramifications of the brain's nerve cells?

---

* The synapse indicates a functional zone of contact that is established between two neurons or a neuron and another cell (muscular cells, sensory receivers).

† Beta-amyloid protein is a peptide consisting of forty to forty-two amino acids.

In short, the production of testosterone decreases with age in men and women. Androgens act by several well-identified, different mechanisms. Male hormones have the following functions:

- Stimulate growth, ramification, and insulation of nervous fibers
- Prevent cerebral arteries from being affected by sclerosis
- Avoid the production of β-amyloid protein and its consequent deposition in the brain
- Prevention of Alzheimer's disease from the appearance of the first symptoms, and even before, when the production of male hormones is insufficient

Simple proportioning of testosterone in the blood is not enough to establish the diagnosis. A detailed study of androgen production is essential in each person (man or woman) who has Alzheimer's disease. Biochemical detection of the deficits and their therapeutic corrections are quite determining, particularly at the beginning of the disease. Treatment of androgen deficits is safe (chapter 31). Clinical and biological studies conducted in this direction will give positive results very quickly.

Summary

Major pharmaceutical companies have abandoned research on molecules that did not provide any effects on Alzheimer's disease.

The pharmaceutical problem is the fact that the pharmaceutical industry is interested in the final phase of the illness, whereas this treatment begins tens of years before.

Alzheimer's disease is a global disaster that can affect anyone. Interesting studies have already given some indications about testosterone and Alzheimer's disease [1–16]. Their results will be better understood through new research that considers the following:

- Studies generally look at blood testosterone levels without regard to blood dihydrotestosterone levels.
- At the same time, dihydrotestosterone is a significant source of androgen hormone production.
- Hormonal studies are concerned with blood testosterone levels and not with the total and daily production of this hormone and of its precursors and its metabolites.
- Studies on sex hormones that do not consider dihydrotestosterone and testosterone production as well as all androgen precursors and metabolites, compared to the female hormone production chain, are therefore incomplete and challenging to interpret—even unusable.
- It seems to me that it is consequently logical to carry out urgently those new studies. There is no reason to wait.

28

Stroke

Stroke is a sudden neurological deficit of vascular origin caused by infarction or hemorrhage of the brain. Fifteen percent of strokes are hemorrhagic, generally causing hemiplegia. Signs are variable according to the localization of the cerebral lesion. This kind of stroke is usually the consequence of sudden arterial hypertension, having produced a rupture of a blood vessel wall. This incident is sometimes the result of a poorly adapted anticoagulant treatment. Eighty percent of strokes are ischemic. Diabetes and hypertension are the principal causes because these diseases lead to a thickening of the walls of small cerebral arteries until their occlusion. The lack of contribution of oxygen causes the death of the nerve cells. The probability of having an ischemic stroke increases with age.

Prevalence

In the United States, there are 795,000 strokes each year, of which 610,000 represent a first brain attack, and 185,000 cases constitute relapses. A person has an attack every forty seconds [1].

Strokes are a pandemic, according to the World Health Organization (WHO). An increased incidence will lead from 16 million in 2005 to 23 million in 2030. Mortality from stroke will increase from 5.7 to 12 million in the same period [2].

Symptoms

Apparent symptoms are the loss of mobility of an arm or a leg, deviation of the mouth, and paralysis of half of the body. Other symptoms, such as difficulty expressing oneself or eye troubles, are alarming signals.

Take care of headaches. They can mean imminent cerebral hemorrhage caused by ignored hypertension, where no neurological symptoms exist.

Mortality Rate

In 2011, stroke was the twentieth-leading cause of death in the United States. As noted, a person dies of a stroke every four minutes [1]. Twenty to 30 percent of the patients having strokes die in the first three months, 45 percent die in six months, and 70 percent die in five years.

The cost of strokes in the United States reaches $34 billion a year [3], including medical benefits, drugs, and work incapacities. In Canada, the annual cost of strokes is $3.6 billion.

Ischemic stroke does not occur by chance. It is generally the consequence of the obstruction of a cerebral artery by a narrowing of its diameter or by a clot, which destroys cerebral tissue. Stroke caused by aging is the result of the interaction all the degradations of the organism described in this book:

- Fatty untreated diabetes (chapter 8)
- Triglyceride and cholesterol excess (chapter 9)
- Atheroma (chapter 9)
- Excess weight and obesity (chapter 10)
- Arterial rigidity and arteriosclerosis (chapter 12)
- Anemia (chapter 13)
- Thick blood (chapter 14)

- Untreated hypertension (chapter 15)
- Coronary disease and myocardial infarction (chapter 16)
- Degeneration of connective tissue (chapter 17)
- Degeneration of the nervous system (chapter 27)

In other words, a woman of age seventy who measures 1.70 meters in height, weighs 150 pounds, has a healthy blood pressure of 12/8, and has a cholesterol level of 150 mg/100 mL of plasma has little chance of having a stroke in the immediate future. In contrast, a woman of seventy who measures 1.70 meters in height, weighs 250 pounds, has a blood pressure of 16/10, and has a cholesterol level of 260 mg/100 mL of plasma is likely to have a stroke or a heart infarct in the immediate future.

Stroke is a medical emergency that requires immediate action and medical care. The speed with which the victim of a stroke arrives at a hospital offering specialized services for acute stroke determines the chance of survival with few or no incapacities. The public generally ignores the characteristics of a stroke and the importance of detecting, in time, the risk factor preceding the stroke: hypertension.

Stroke and Dementia

Vascular dementia is a disorder caused by multiple small cerebral vascular incidents in the brain that generate a variety of cognitive symptoms, including memory disorders.

Strokes constitute the first cause of a physical handicap acquired in the adult and the second cause of dementia, after Alzheimer's disease.

Part IV

Revitalize Your Body

29

The Anti-Aging Hormone

There are phenomena whose causes and symptoms are apparent. A drop in blood pressure caused by external bleeding, with its spectacular manifestation, is understood more quickly because the reason is simple: a trauma. If the cause is internal bleeding, it is a little more complicated; it is necessary to seek the organ responsible for the bleeding. Immediate treatment consists of a blood transfusion, but the bleeding should be stopped at the same time through wound closure and possible removal of the diseased organ.

A short return through time will show how a disease can exist for centuries without people being aware of it. In the case of this disease, billions of human beings died prematurely without knowing why.

Before the Second World War, infectious diseases still caused devastation in the West. Archaeological discoveries showed that this specific disease existed since antiquity. The remains of bodies showed inflammatory tumors in all organs. Tubercular lesions were also found in Egyptian mummies.

Aristotle had already recognized the contagiousness of the disease, and Hippocrates, noting the extreme exhaustion of the patients, had given the name *phthisis* to this mysterious disease.

The bloody sputum of the Lady to the Camellias (*La Dame aux camélias*) remained famous, and it was a tragedy of ignorance.

In 1819, Laennec, an exceptional doctor, recognized the unicity of the disease. In his treatise on the use of the stethoscope, he affirmed that all tubercular lesions from the lung transformed into a huge abscess, then destroyed the kidneys, and that the deformed bones producing hunchbacks resulted from the same disease.

This theory was the object of controversy for more than fifty years; most doctors could not see the relationship between hunchbacks and bloody sputum. Great outdoors and rest were the only treatments. The cause of the disease was unknown. Deaths amounted to millions.

In 1882, Koch described the bacillus responsible for the tubercular lesions, but lives were not spared because of it. It was necessary to find the remedy, which took sixty-two more years. In 1944, Waksman discovered streptomycin, a solution against tuberculosis. But it is essential to have the antibiotic—one can still die of the disease today, most often in the Third World, due to a lack of information and money.

Closer to our time, researchers discovered the secrets of AIDS quickly despite the diversity of its symptoms: lung infection, cerebral abscesses, and cancer of the skin known as *Kaposi's sarcoma*. Thanks to the power of scientific research, the cause of this affliction was found quickly by Luc Montagnier and his team, who isolated the responsible virus. Several drugs are already able to knock back the disease. At the beginning of the epidemic, AZT was used, and now quadruple therapy is used to delay the progression of the virus. Interferons cured certain cases of Kaposi's sarcoma. Knowledge about this pathology progresses unceasingly, and one can hope for the control of it in years to come to finish this plague by the end of the twentieth century.

A disaster just as frightening threatens humanity. It exists everywhere and causes devastation: aging diseases. Such diseases are omnipresent in different forms that do not seem to have any relationship among them. And yet, why, when men get old, is there suddenly this blow that unrelentingly leads them toward decrepitude, passing the second half of their lives with disease and suffering? Why are they generally in good health before age forty? If a basic principle exists that explains good health, that is what is lacking when the body starts to become degraded. Some will say it is genetic, but everything is genetic. That is not an adequate explanation.

And what if aging begins with the incapacity to secrete the hormone of life: testosterone?

From 1945 until now, medicine has triumphed in many fields, thanks to a whole panoply of drugs and techniques, increasingly sophisticated, so that woman's life expectancy has risen to 86.8 years today in the country where men live longest: Japan.

The median age is indeed progressing—but by keeping people barely alive, isolated in their small rooms, stuck in their armchairs, or confined to the bed.

The diseases of aging can be defeated only when the cause is defined, and a remedy is found.

And what if the cause of sexual aging is the same as that which starts general aging?

In a young woman, the ovaries produce around two hundred micrograms of testosterone (more than female hormones) daily. This quantity acts locally in the body with amounts in the picograms (thousandths of a billionth of a gram).

The genitals use only one small part of this production. The most significant quantity of secreted testosterone is used by all organs of the human body that need some amount to maintain and regenerate their protein structures, without which no life is possible.

Consequently, two hundred million picograms are necessary daily to make the body function and to maintain organs in a good state.

This fact explains a lot of diseases that occur after age forty. They appear according to individuals' unique biology and worsen unrelentingly with time.

The following disorders appear in the woman with androgenic disease of menopause according to a particular disorder; general weaknesses are also common.

Masculine Genitalia Problems

- Pain during intercourse
- Urgency to urinate
- Cystitis
- Incontinence
- Reduction in libido

General Diseases of Aging

- Excess of weight
- Obesity
- Urination troubles: cystitis, urgencies, incontinence
- Depression, poor image of oneself, irritability, melancholy, suicidal tendency, incapacity to act
- Migraine headaches
- Incapacity to react to stress
- Intestinal distension
- Osteoarthritis (shoulder, knee, hip, spinal column)
- Brittleness of articular ligaments
- Osteoporosis (osseous brittleness, fractures)

- Muscular brittleness
- Hypertension
- Angina pectoris
- Myocardial infarction
- Arteriosclerosis
- Varicose veins
- Hemorrhoids
- Varicose ulcers
- Gangrene
- Anemia
- Thick blood
- Arterial or venous thrombosis
- A rise in blood cholesterol (especially "bad" cholesterol)
- An increase in blood triglycerides
- Diabetes
- Wrinkles
- Inadequate filtration of the kidneys, leading to uremia
- Immunizing deficit, predisposing to cancers
- Vision trouble
- Hearing disorders
- Loose teeth

At first sight, these numerous diseases and symptoms do not have any relationship among them. Attempting to find their link may seem deceptive.

A first reflection is essential: Do these symptoms or groups of symptoms or diseases exist? The answer is yes. Anyone can observe that.

Then, are these gathered phenomena the expression of aging? The answer is yes. Let us consider older men. They present these apparent disorders.

The third point is essential to this reflection. A common link connects all these phenomena: they can be caused in whole or in part by a lack of male hormones. It is a fact shown by many scientific studies published over many years. Continuation of the reasoning comes logically. If the hormone is missing, why not give it to those who show a decrease in androgen production?

But does this hormone exist in the form of drugs? The answer is, yet again, yes. Testosterone has been available since 1936 in the form of intramuscular injections.

We have the symptoms, the disease, and the antidote. We should not be losing a moment.

The phenomena of aging appear successively. They appear as symptoms treated by traditional medicine. But each degenerative event can cause others that cause still other symptoms.

It is like a Russian doll, where each doll hides a smaller one, and so on. One can imagine a similar system where one puppet would be replaced by a chicken and another by an egg.

Each chicken would hide a smaller egg, which, in turn, would conceal a smaller chicken. One cannot escape the fundamental questions: Where does the chicken come from, and where does the egg originate? Regarding aging diseases, the problem becomes more complicated. The chickens and the eggs are different colors. It follows a seemingly inextricable tangle, a labyrinth from which it is possible to leave only thanks to a guiding thread (*le fil d'Ariane*). This thread is the male hormone.

Excess weight and obesity involve the overloading of bones and joint articulations, which wear more quickly, accelerating the appearance of osteoarthritis. At the same time, the body mass needs more blood flooding, and the blood pressure rises automatically. I will mention just three complications with this example for ease of presentation.

First, it is the overload of the organism that causes, for mechanical reasons, the wear of joint articulations and the increase in blood pressure. Second, a lack of male hormones causes the accumulation of fats and an excess of weight. Third, the walls of the arteries become rigid from a lack of male hormones, thus causing hypertension that worsens with overweight.

The same phenomenon occurs in fragile joint articulations. Deprived of male hormones, they crush more easily when there is an overload.

To avoid degeneration and to maintain the human body in good health, it is necessary to act on all the pathological factors simultaneously.

For technical reasons, mesterolone is the right anti-aging hormone, as we will see later (chapter 31).

30

Control Your Aging

Sexual aging and the general aging of the human body are syndromes. To treat a body without taking its state into account is not enough because, in this case, there is no solution. The general condition of the human body must be the object of individual attention.

Beyond age forty, the body is often more destroyed than we think. To the observer who can see (it is enough to one's open eyes), the degenerative transformations are already apparent. If you are over forty, don't you believe yourself to be sick? Look attentively at yourself naked in a mirror. Observe your face, your chest, your belly, your profile, your arms, and your legs. Compare this image with one of your photographs in a swimsuit between the ages of twenty and twenty-five. The differences are the result of aging.

Is your face the same one? Do you recognize yourself? Do you accept the pasted-on look, with its solidified features, inexpressive mimicry, and sad glance?

Does your well-developed thorax allow full or reduced breathing? Does it allow only weak, superficial breathing? Are you the same size as you were at twenty-five?

Does your belly resemble a stratospheric balloon more and more? Are your buttocks made of fat or muscles? What became of your arms and your legs?

What is the state of your skin? Did you lose your pilosity? Are your nails hard or breakable? Are your breasts prominent? Did you get shorter by one or several centimeters? Are your shoulders arched? Is your back aligned?

Now go to the silhouettes of the regressive woman shown in the figure 19, page 108. At age twenty-five, the silhouette represents the woman at the peak of her development. The profiles at thirty, forty, and fifty-five years of age are all degenerative. Locate your silhouette. Do not be afraid. Even if you correspond to the drawing of fifty-five years, you can go the opposite way, successively passing by the silhouettes of forty and thirty years. In the best case, while working on yourself, you will be able to reach the profile of twenty-five years.

The ideal is to react quickly and not to enter the extreme forms of degeneration.

Visible damage outside is the expression of devastation inside the body, in all organs, including the brain.

The damage caused by a lack of rest, immobility, self-destruction by tobacco use, and unhealthy food is considerable. Control of these harmful factors is essential and constitutes a precondition to the biochemical control of the body after age forty. Smokers, the sedentary or overly stressed, alcoholics, and the obese have a short life.

Early sexual pain, depression, and micturition problems lead many women to go for consultations. They hope for a miracle cure to solve all their problems. But doctors are not aware that male hormones can be missing in women.

Furthermore, to biologically maintain and prolong the existence of an older body is practically unrealizable in the absence of a healthful lifestyle. At the risk of upsetting some candidates for longevity, I tell them from the start: do not smoke, arrange your working time, and do exercise.

People are what they eat and what they drink. At one level, drinking and eating involve something pleasant and convivial. In terms of longevity, food is essential; alcohol and fat make a mess of male hormones.

Chronic alcoholism gradually destroys the liver; patients with cirrhosis have perturbed sex hormones. The disease of alcoholism destroys the integrity of the nervous system and the testicles. Under these conditions, alcoholics are bad candidates for hormonal replacement therapy.

Excess fat is also damaging. A more massive silhouette is the result of the fatty degeneration of the body. The overload starts with the first extra pound. It is common to note overloads of twenty to forty pounds and more. On this subject, did you calculate your body mass index (BMI)? (If not, see chapter 10.)

Fat has the property of collecting and neutralizing male hormones. To ensure effective hormonal treatment, it is necessary, at all costs, to eliminate unnecessary fat by controlling your diet. If you have a weight problem, learn the energy value of food and the various dietetic methods by consulting the many books that cover this issue. If necessary, do not hesitate to consult your doctor. The goal is to reach the weight you were between twenty and twenty-five years old (if you did not have a weight problem at that age).

A simple blood test is sometimes enough to make the diagnosis of hormonal insufficiency. A complete study of hormonal production is often necessary. Levels of sex hormones at a given time provide the hormonal profile that is ideal in women from age twenty to twenty-five, not presenting any organic or degenerative sexual problem. These are the biological conditions that are necessary to restore one's youth as much as possible.

31

Hormonal Treatment

First, do no harm

—Hippocrates, 410 BC

Before beginning treatment, it is necessary to understand its mechanism. Twenty-first-century medicine is a scientific medicine, without which there is no *Ageless Woman* in good health. This book is only an introduction to therapy. The reader needs to be aware of it. It starts now.

Treatments That Harm Androgenic Disease of Menopause

- Hormone replacement therapy (HRT)
- Bioidentical HRT

Hormone Replacement Therapy (HRT)

Madness is always to do the same thing,

waiting for different results.

—Albert Einstein

HRT is any form of hormone therapy wherein the patient, in the course of medical treatment, receives hormones, either to supplement a lack of naturally occurring hormones or to substitute other hormones for naturally occurring hormones.

HRT for menopause comes from the idea that the treatment may prevent the discomfort caused by diminished circulating estrogen and progesterone hormones or, in the case of the surgically or prematurely menopausal, that it may prolong life and reduce the incidence of dementia. The main types of hormones involved are estrogens, progesterone, or progestins, and sometimes, testosterone presented as "treatment" rather than therapy. All those "treatments" are wrong.

Replacement with estrogen and progesterone is a fatal error because these hormones are no longer needed and are even dangerous after menopause.

Even testosterone replacement is wrong because testosterone is a precursor of estradiol, the proliferative hormone.

US Food and Drug Administration (FDA) Warnings about HRT

Booklet from FDA about HRT

Office of Women's Health

"Medicines to Help You" (pdf format)

Download:

http://www.georgesdebled.org/menopause medicines to help you.pdf

Menopause

Some women choose to treat their menopause symptoms with hormone medicines. The booklet of the FDA lists some necessary information about the FDA-approved hormone medicines for menopause.

There are different types of hormone medicines used during and after menopause:

- Estrogen-Only Medicines
- Progestin-Only Medicines
- Combination Estrogen and Progestin Medicines
- Combination Estrogen and Other Medicines

According to the FDA, Do not take hormone therapy if you:

- have problems with vaginal bleeding
- have or have had certain cancers such as breast cancer or uterine cancer
- have or have had a blood clot, stroke, or heart attack
- have a bleeding disorder
- have liver disease
- have allergic reactions to hormone medicine
- Have had a stroke or heart attack
- Have liver problems
- Have severe reactions to estrogen medicines
- Think you are pregnant
- Have or have had blood clots in the legs or lungs

According to the FDA, the sides effects are as follows:

Less Serious, Common Side Effects

- Headaches
- Painful or tender breasts
- Vaginal spotting

- Stomach cramps/bloating
- Nausea and vomiting
- Hair loss
- Fluid retention
- Vaginal yeast infection
- Muscle spasms
- Diarrhea
- Upset stomach/stomach pain
- Throat pain
- Dizziness
- Neck Pain

The severe side effects are

- Stroke
- Endometrial cancer in women who still have their uterus and who do not use progestin with estrogen-only medicines
- Heart attack
- Blood clots
- Breast cancer
- Dementia in women 65 years and older
- Gallbladder disease or high triglyceride (cholesterol) levels that could lead to problems with your pancreas
- Liver problems
- Vision loss caused by a blood clot in the eye
- High blood pressure
- Severe allergic reactions

These side effects are frightening, and the FDA booklet does not list all of the side effects and warnings for each hormone medicine.

Is Bioidentical Hormone Replacement Therapy a Solution?

Again, the best advice comes from the FDA. See the content in the FDA pamphlet "Bioidenticals: Sorting Myths from Facts."

Estriol in the US

Also spelled oestriol, this steroid is a weak estrogen. It is one of three major endogenous estrogens, the others being estradiol and estrone.

FDA has not approved any drug containing estriol. The safety and effectiveness of estriol are unknown. "No data have been submitted to FDA that demonstrate that estriol is safe and effective," according to Daniel Shames, M.D., a senior official in the FDA office that oversees reproductive products.

Brand names for estriol

A variety of brand names market estriol throughout the world, including Aacifemine, Blissel, Colpogyn, Elinol, Estriel, Estriol, Estriosalbe, Estrokad, Evalon, Gelistrol, Gydrelle, Gynasan, Gynest, Incurin (veterinary), OeKolp, Oestro-Gynaedron, Orgestriol, Ortho-Gynest, Ovesterin, Ovestin, Ovestinon, Ovestrion, Pausanol, Physiogine, Sinapause, Synapause, Trophicreme, and Vacidox, among others.

Future of Hormonal Replacement Therapy and Estetrol

Research is currently evaluating the interest in replacing the natural hormones of the hormonal cycle—estradiol and progesterone—with a combination of estetrol and progesterone [1]. One may wonder why it would be necessary to replace hormones that have become useless because they are hormones that control ovulation when it exists. What is the use of these hormones when there are no eggs? And with a uterus that no longer serves a purpose?

In recent years, pharmacological trials have been undertaken to determine whether it is useful for women to take estetrol after menopause. Because estetrol has a **proliferative effect** on the structures of the uterus, administration of estetrol for twenty-eight days also requires the taking of a progestin for two weeks to reduce the proliferation of the mucosa that covers the inner lining of the uterus. A study published in June 2017 in *Menopause* prudently supports the further investigation of estetrol as a candidate for HRT [2].

> A "less harmful treatment" is not necessarily the right treatment.

Premature Menopause or Early Menopause

Women undergoing premature or early menopause experience the rapid loss of estrogen and other ovarian hormones. It happens either following bilateral removal of ovaries or because of primary ovarian insufficiency.

Long-term consequences of premature or early menopause include adverse effects on cognition, mood, the cardiovascular system, bone, and sexual health, as well as an increased risk of early mortality.

The use of "classic hormone therapy" has been shown to lessen some, although not all, of these risks. Therefore, multiple medical societies recommend providing hormone therapy at least until the natural age of menopause.

Women who experience premature menopause (before age forty) or early menopause (between forty and forty-five) experience an increased risk of overall mortality, cardiovascular disease, neurological disease, psychiatric disorders, osteoporosis, and other sequelae. The risk of adverse outcomes increases with earlier age at the time of menopause.

Several departments of the Women's Health Clinic of the Mayo Clinic in Rochester, New York, confirm that estrogen alone does not prevent all long-term consequences and suggest that other hormonal mechanisms are likely involved [3]. Estradiol and progesterone-only treatments intend to produce a regular menstrual cycle. If there is no uterus, those hormones are not necessary. If menopause is premature, in the presence of a uterus, it may be hazardous to take estradiol and progesterone compositions [4]. However, testosterone and dihydrotestosterone remain necessary for life.

Women who experience premature menopause or early menopause and are treated with mesterolone will have the same future as any woman correctly treated for the common problems of menopause.

The dogma of estrogen and progesterone replacement after menopause is so entrenched in the mind-set of physicians that despite warnings from the FDA, one in two physicians still prescribes these "treatments."

Conclusion of the FDA

> According to the FDA, all treatments that include estrogen, progesterone, or progestin alone or combined may cause dangerous side effects. The list of such effects is impressive.

HRT with any component of any estrogen plus any progestogen will lead to failure because, after menopause, those hormones are not necessary anymore. The "classic hormone replacement" proposed so far still involves the same thinking: the dangerous replacement of unnecessary hormones and the non-replacement of vital hormones.

What about Estradiol and Progesterone Production in Menopause?

Estradiol is a proliferative hormone needed to build the egg's "nest" in the uterus during the first part of the menstrual cycle.

Progesterone is the specific hormone of the second part of the menstrual cycle. It is a hormone that relaxes the musculature of the uterus to prepare it for pregnancy. In the absence of progesterone, there may be contractions of uterine musculature that cause miscarriage.

During the entire menstrual cycle, the ovaries produce testosterone in large amounts. It is a hormone that contracts the muscles of the uterus. The massive production of progesterone counterbalances this contracting action during the second part of the menstrual cycle.

Pregnancy begins with a fertilized egg, and the secretion of progesterone then increases considerably until the end of the pregnancy.

When menstruation stops around age fifty, the estradiol–progesterone program is no longer needed because there is no more egg to fertilize. Then why prescribe estrogen and progesterone when the human reproductive program is over? From where does this idea come?

HRT for menopause emerged after the production of the contraceptive pill in the 1950s. Women who take the contraceptive pill arrive progressively at the age of menopause when the production of estrogen and progesterone ceases. Some women experience hot flashes or night sweats or are affected by dryness and vaginal fragility. Doctors in this era thought that it was necessary to continue the menstrual cycle artificially by using combinations of estradiol and progestins to alleviate these discomforts. The idea gradually changed to preventing certain diseases of aging. HRT was born. But this was a misunderstanding of the problem, as demonstrated later by the Women's Health Initiative (WHI).

The WHI Study

The US National Institutes of Health sponsored the WHI study, a fifteen-year project involving over 161,000 women aged fifty to seventy-nine. The WHI represents one of the most definitive, far-reaching programs of research on women's health ever undertaken in the United States (see www.whi.org). The first HRT study, "Risks and Benefits of Estrogen Plus Progestin in Healthy Postmenopausal Women," published the results in 2002 in the *Journal of American Medical Association* [4]. Conclusions about this randomized clinical trial of significant scale relating to 16,608 older women from fifty to seventy-nine years of age treated with progestin (2.5 mg of medroxyprogesterone acetate) and estrogens (0.625 mg of combined estrogens, "equine") were reported (see the following table).

The study was to proceed until 2005. However, it stopped after a 5.2-year-average follow-up on July 9, 2002, but continued the treatment containing estrogens alone among women with a prior hysterectomy.
The WHI Estrogen Alone (E-Alone) trial assessed the health benefits and risks of estrogen use in healthy postmenopausal women.

Women Taking Estrogen Plus Progestin Relative to Placebo
Stroke rates increased by 41 percent
Coronary heart disease (CHD) events increased by 29 percent
Venous thromboembolism (VTEs) were twofold greater
Total cardiovascular disease increased by 22 percent
Breast cancer increased by 26 percent

According to Rossouw and al. (2002) [4].

In the WHI E-Alone Trial, 10,739 women with a prior hysterectomy, aged fifty to seventy-nine years, were assigned to take either estrogen alone (conjugated estrogens) or inactive (placebo) study pills. The

National Institutes of Health stopped the E-Alone Trial ahead of schedule in February 2004, primarily because of increased stroke risk for women taking the pills with estrogen alone.

Over six million women took menopause drugs before the WHI study [4]. Other publications [5–8] pointed out their links to breast cancer.

The WHI found that the risks of menopausal hormone therapy (HRT) outweighed the benefits for asymptomatic women. After this study in 2002, about half of gynecologists in the United States continued to believe that the traditional HRT benefited women's health. The pharmaceutical industry has supported the publication of articles supporting HRT in medical journals for marketing purposes [9]. Yet, women using the medicines have had a 26 percent higher risk of breast cancer.

Class Actions in the United States

Three Nevada women who contracted breast cancer after taking menopause drugs were awarded millions in a 2007 case. The amount was the largest to be upheld on appeal among thousands of HRT suits. Since 2011 in the United States, pharmaceutical companies have faced more than ten thousand claims from former users of menopause drugs. Billions were set aside by pharmacies to resolve complaints about HRT medicine.

Collapsed "Classic" HRT

There has been a decline in new cases of breast cancer since the use of HRT has collapsed in countries such as France, the United States, Canada, and Great Britain. It is therefore challenging to continue to argue that the increased risk of breast cancer observed with HRT was due solely to a "promoter effect" on cancer cells already present in the breast that would have simply revealed a latent tumor. This is especially the case because many studies, not just the WHI, have shown an increased risk of breast cancer with HRT.

In 2017, a review was done by the Department of Endocrine and Breast Surgery at the First Affiliated Hospital of Chongqing Medical University, Chongqing, China. The meta-analysis concluded that the current use of estrogen-alone therapy or estrogen-plus-progestin therapy is associated with an elevated risk of breast cancer [10].

That same year, at the Annual Meeting of the North American Menopause Society in Philadelphia, it was emphasized that there were significantly more significant side effects with pellet versus FDA-approved HRT. Women treated with estradiol and testosterone pellet therapy experienced six times the number of adverse side effects, including abnormal uterine bleeding and subsequent hysterectomy, according to findings from a retrospective cohort study [11].

Ovaries of Healthy Women Secrete More Testosterone Than Estradiol Each Day

The ovaries produce more or less testosterone after menopause, depending on particular conditions (chapter 1, [4]).

Because the physiological production of testosterone is significant in healthy women, doctors thought it was useful to replace this third hormone in menopausal women as well, mainly in menopausal women deprived of sexual desire.

We can first ask ourselves what creates the sexual desire of women. Treating this lack of excitement with testosterone is illogical because testosterone is not the real sex hormone—dihydrotestosterone—that is necessary to maintain the normal functions of the masculine genitalia.

In 2010, regarding testosterone therapy to combat reduced libido in women, Rosemary Basson, professor of sexual medicine in the Department of Psychiatry at British Columbia University, Vancouver, Canada, concluded:

> We do not have evidence of low androgen activity in women with low sexual libido, nor studies of testosterone supplementation in women with specific sexual disorders, where criteria for the diagnosis of the disorder are more robust. Long-term risks of testosterone supplementation are unknown. [12]

We should first define female desire. What is desire? It seems hazardous to want to medicalize female desire, which is not to be confused with the sexual pleasure derived from a woman's masculine sexual organs. It is not easy for a woman to seek sexual pleasure when she suffers from genital pain that comes from progressive atrophy of her sexual organs when dihydrotestosterone is missing.

The FDA and Testosterone Replacement Therapy in Women

The FDA cautions against the prescription of testosterone products. They are indicated *only for men* who have low testosterone levels caused *by certain medical conditions* (FDA Safety Announcement 03-03-2015).

Extensive long-term treatments of testosterone in women may prove to show harm rather than therapy. Indeed, testosterone is not a sex hormone. It is a precursor that is necessary to make estradiol—the female proliferative hormone. Thus, a testosterone gel or patch applied to a woman is likely to produce the same long-term problems as those described in the WHI study (see the previous discussion). North America does not approve of testosterone therapy for women. Once again, the FDA is prudent and well-advised in this regard.

Understanding Hormones Secreted by Ovaries and Sexual Receptors

Each day, the ovaries produce androgens. This poorly understood hormone production is the fundamental problem of menopause.

During the menstrual cycle, the ovaries secrete estradiol, progesterone, and testosterone directly. Daily testosterone production is higher than estradiol production because estradiol comes from the transformation of testosterone. A significant amount of testosterone is also converted immediately into dihydrotestosterone by the masculine genitalia and androgen receptors of women.

Testosterone is not a male hormone, strictly speaking. The confusion comes from the fact that testosterone is an "androgen." The word *androgen* signifies, according to *Webster's New World College Dictionary*: a type of natural or artificial steroid that acts as a male sex hormone.

According to the *American Heritage Dictionary of the English Language*, the word *androgen* signifies a steroid hormone, such as testosterone or androsterone, that controls the development and maintenance of masculine characteristics.

Testosterone must be converted into dihydrotestosterone by an enzyme, 5α-reductase. Men who are deprived of 5α-reductase do not have masculine structures. They look like women, but their chromosomes are male (XY). They are known as *hairless women* and are generally beautiful. Because they secrete a large amount of testosterone, these individuals can have plasma levels of testosterone of around 1,500 nanograms per hundred milliliters of plasma, a higher level than *the most "male" man can produce* (a normal young man generally secretes 700 to 1,000 nanograms at age twenty).

The word *androgen* introduces confusion in defining the role of *each androgenic hormone.* Dehydroepiandrosterone (DHEA), androstenedione, androsterone, testosterone, dihydrotestosterone, and other synthetic hormones are considered as *androgens* or *androgenic hormones*. The general term *androgen* does not explain the specific action of each molecule.

It is impossible to understand medical treatment by using the word *androgen* to represent several molecules that have different biological actions. For example, DHEA is freely available in US drugstores. This *androgenic molecule* is transformed by the body, in varying degrees, into testosterone and estradiol, which have opposed biological effects.

Thus, properly speaking, testosterone is not an "androgen." It is a precursor of the real androgen—dihydrotestosterone—as well as a precursor of estradiol, the real female hormone. It is surprising to note that a discussion of dihydrotestosterone is generally absent from all scientific studies concerning androgen replacement in women.

Testosterone is also a specific anabolic hormone that controls all protein structures of the body in men and women. The body degenerates in its absence, leading to diseases of aging diseases.

The decrease in testosterone production is manifested very clearly, at the beginning of aging, in a reduction in the production of its active sex hormone metabolite—dihydrotestosterone. Therefore, sexual aging, which precedes general aging, is a warning signal. Indeed, the output of testosterone continuously decreases by producing degeneration of all structures of the body.

Essential Hormones for Androgenic Disease of Menopause

For more than fifty years, doctors have considered that hot flashes, difficulty sleeping, feeling anxious, and depression are the result of a lack of estrogens, progesterone, or both. Those symptoms are the result of another pathogenesis.

In one case, a sixty-nine-year-old postmenopausal woman presented with several months of worsening hair growth on the face, neck, chin, torso, and arms, requiring shaving. Laboratory testing revealed markedly elevated testosterone levels (160 nanograms/100 mL; normal is ± 50 nanograms/100 mL). There was no ovarian or adrenal abnormality. She started a suppressive treatment of testosterone that resulted in a dramatic decline in testosterone levels. *The woman reported significant "hot flashes," difficulty sleeping, anxiety, and depression secondary to treatment, and the patient discontinued leuprolide therapy three months after initiation.* After stopping the suppressive treatment of testosterone, she reported being generally in good spirits [13].

This extraordinary story points to evidence and begs several questions.

Evidence

- The ovaries may secrete testosterone after menopause.

- There is female individuality in hormone production, requiring singular treatment in each woman.
- This explains why some women have menopausal problems and others do not.
- It also explains why symptoms can appear sooner or later, depending on singular hormonal production that decreases individually.
- Hot flashes, difficulty sleeping, feeling anxious, and depression may be the result of a lack of testosterone production in a woman.
- Hot flashes, difficulty sleeping, feeling anxious, and depression may disappear when natural testosterone production is restored.

Questions

- Should testosterone and dihydrotestosterone be dosed in all postmenopausal women with disorders?
- Should testosterone and dihydrotestosterone be dosed in all women with premature menopause and early menopause who experience disorders?
- Should testosterone and dihydrotestosterone be replaced in postmenopausal women with menopause disorders?
- Are pellets or patches of testosterone safe, knowing that testosterone transforms into **estradiol, the proliferative hormone (increasing the risk of breast cancer)?**
- Should we avoid HRT with estrogens, progesterone, or both, which can be in contradiction with the use of testosterone?
- When and how should androgen replacement proceed if deemed necessary?
- Is there a known safe treatment?

Conclusion

Why prescribe estrogen and progesterone when the human reproductive program is over? And why not prescribe androgens that are no longer secreted—from the same ovaries—after menopause and that are necessary to maintain the normal functions of the masculine genitalia and entire body?

Androgenic menopausal disease is the result of the decreased secretion of testosterone and dihydrotestosterone. It is aggravated by the administration of the conventional treatment called "menopausal treatment" (HRT).

All traditional HRT drugs cause a decrease in the production of testosterone and dihydrotestosterone or the inhibition of hormonal receptors of these androgens.

The madness here is wanting to continually redo HRT for hormones that are no longer necessary, estrogens and progesterone, for the reproduction program. Furthermore, essential hormones for the body (testosterone and dihydrotestosterone) are poorly known and thus ignored and not replaced.

I have even met doctors, highly qualified in their specialty, who fear to prescribe small amounts of mesterolone to women who need it, despite the proof of its deficiency. These same physicians were continuing to take, for themselves, combinations of estrogen and progesterone without fear, neglecting the prudent advice of the FDA. With mesterolone, this confusion is not possible.

> The best way to create androgenic disease of menopause is to take estrogens (all) and progestogens.
>
> Androgenic disease of menopause is a disease of aging.
>
> The fastest and most effective way to induce a disease of aging is not to treat androgenic disease of menopause.
>
> The best way to age a woman quickly is to prescribe a combination of estrogen (all) and progestogens.

Mesterolone Treatment of Androgen Deficiencies in Women

Birth of the Concept

At the beginning of the 1970s, I realized that the hormonal aspect of sexual disorders was unknown. I had just obtained my qualification of *agrégé de l'enseignement supérieur en sciences urologiques.*[*]

Because impotent men were considered "psychopaths," the university education about this pathology was nonexistent. But because they were numerous and complained in similar terms about symptoms or identical groups of symptoms, I considered the situation. It was one of two things: either the hundreds of patients who complained about impotence were insane, and the doctor who diagnosed psychopathy was right, or the patients were right, and it was the doctor who was entirely off. I took the side of the patients and decided to study the problem from the hormonal approach, mainly because the determination of hormone levels was easily achievable by 1974. I realized very quickly that the male hormone levels of older men were decreased, causing, initially, medically reversible impotence or

[*] In Europe, for some disciplines of higher education, such as urology, there is an *agrégation* for the professorship positions called *agrégation de l'enseignement supérieur.*

mechanical impotence by arteriosclerosis when the hormonal deficit had caused its destroying effects. I started to prescribe hormones in quantity, with increasingly convincing results, and to place penile implants surgically in impotent patients whose arteries were blocked, with extremely encouraging results.

I was teaching at Brussels University, the part of the course of urology devoted to andrology. The full professor of urology had fallen ill for a long time, so I proceeded to draw up urology examinations for the students of the third degree in medicine.

The director of the hospital where I worked decided to create a university service specialized in andrology, parallel to the service of urology. As in any pyramidal structure, the chief watched over the service, it being essential for him not to lose power. The hospital depending on the university, along with the "chief," arranged to create a commission with his old friends, sitting behind closed doors, to make a scientific lawsuit against me. What could be better than to institute a special court to bar me at all costs? They declared me insane because I treated and operated on impotence, whereas everyone knew that it was a mental disease. Deemed "crazy," I joined the rows of demented patients (one has the doctor one deserves). Determined to fight to clear up andropause problems, I decided to leave the hospital.

Two years later, after a stormy debate in which it was a question of knowing if a young chief could cohabitate with an old boss, the board of directors of the university granted my resignation, moderately. My career as an associate professor was thus cut short after such a promising beginning!

Meanwhile, I had created, in 1974, a private medical center specializing in andrology, which received more patients increasingly. This private clinic specializing in sexual pathology was probably one of the first, if not the first, in Europe. I had the honor to receive many doctors who had been my medical professors, as well as professors at other universities, whose condition necessitated andrological surgery, specific hormonal treatment with androgens, or both.

The patients flowed into my private clinic. It very quickly became evident that organic impotence was part of a whole—sexual aging being the consequence of a hormonal insufficiency that caused disorders not only of erection but also of ejaculation and prostate diseases.

During the 1970s, I realized that the patients treated with hormones for their sexual aging often said, "I climb better," or "I don't have knee pain anymore." Others said, "I win again when playing tennis," "My joint pains disappeared," "I regained my memory," and "I am not depressed anymore." At the same time, I noted an improvement in blood sugar, cholesterol, and other biological parameters of the blood. Sexual aging and general aging seemed linked by the same cause: the insufficiency of secretion of the sex hormones. They were guide threads able to explain the degeneration of *androgenic disease of andropause*.

At the same time, women consulted for urination problems due to fibrosis of the bladder neck, similar to prostate atrophy in men. They also had similar symptoms as men, mainly sexual difficulties, urination problems, depression, and signs of diseases of aging. Women had a condition like that of men—androgenic disease of andropause—that, in this case, was *androgenic disease of menopause*: same causes, same effects. Treatment with mesterolone was the solution, with the doses needed being less for women.

Oral administration of mesterolone in amounts between five and ten milligrams per day, and even twenty-five milligrams for a short period, constitutes the specific treatment. However, each treatment is *unique* for each woman after a complete biological checkup.

If there is no symptom, there is no disease. If there is no disease, no *curative* treatment is necessary.

Mesterolone is a hormone prescribed for men to compensate for lack of production of androgens. Used in men since 1967, it was henceforth in the public domain. Its manufacturing technique is known. No harmfulness has been described to date.

Before menopause, a woman secretes 0.2 milligrams of testosterone (= 200 micrograms or 200,000 nanograms or 200,000,000 picograms) on each day of the cycle.

Mesterolone is a safe molecule that has been in use since the 1960s. Its molecular properties are those of dihydrotestosterone.

Mesterolone makes it possible to supplement weak androgen production. Currently, it requires traditional compounding.

Why Is Mesterolone the Treatment for Androgen Deficiencies in Women?

Mesterolone does not transform into estradiol—the proliferative hormone (contrary to testosterone). Its methyl radical inserted on carbon 1 of the testosterone confers this property.

At physiological doses, mesterolone does not influence the secretion of the pituitary gland so that the production of luteinizing hormone (LH) is not modified (contrary to testosterone).

Mesterolone prescribed in small amounts adds its effects to those of testosterone secreted by the body.

With the prescribed physiological pharmacological amounts, doping is impossible, as is overdose. Mesterolone is prescribed orally in amounts varying between approximately five and ten milligrams per day, and even twenty-five milligrams per day for a short period. The secretion of LH by the pituitary gland is not severe (contrary to testosterone).

The molecular structure of mesterolone has characteristics of dihydrotestosterone. It is active on the masculine sex organs of women (clitoris, labia majora, and bladder neck) and brain tissue (preventing Alzheimer's disease; see chapter 27, [13]).

Mesterolone can be prescribed alone. The treatment covers all indications for androgens in women.

Mesterolone, Testosterone, and Dihydrotestosterone

The molecular structure of mesterolone confers unique benefits:

- Mesterolone has properties like those of testosterone.
- Mesterolone has features like those of dihydrotestosterone.

Nonexistent Risks of Virilism with Mesterolone Treatment

Treatment of androgen deficiency simply consists of replacing missing secretions of testosterone **and dihydrotestosterone**. Mesterolone properties allow that. In this case, the woman finds only her former physiological state and prevents the disastrous consequences described throughout this book. Mesterolone used in small amounts allows that.

Virilism, secondary to an excessive administration of mesterolone, is the consequence of doping, which should be avoided in all cases. Virilism does not exist at physiological doses.

About Mesterolone in Women

It was not possible to publish these conclusions before because the consequences of menopause were classically understood as the result of a lack of estradiol and progesterone. This polluted concept is still considered as a "dogma" by doctors in general. Even more, the import and prescription of mesterolone are not possible in the United States. Manufacturers have reserved mesterolone as a treatment only for men. From 1998, and ten years after the first conclusions of the WHI study in 2002, my colleagues and I studied the beneficial action of mesterolone on menopaused women. Our study was possible in Europe, where mesterolone is available under traditional compounding. I disclosed for the first time, in a 2015 medical congress and a medical review [14], the conclusions of the study on mesterolone treatment for androgen deficiencies in women, which is the real solution for women with androgen defects before and after menopause.

Conclusion

Androgenic disease of menopause is a clinical entity with a specific cause, specific consequences, and a specific treatment. It is the consequence of a failure of androgen production (testosterone and dihydrotestosterone) that needs treatment. Since 1998, the treatment of *androgenic disease of menopause* has been successful and without any side effects.

With the help of governments and manufacturers, exhaustive studies will be made to specify the parameters of mesterolone treatment. Treatment of androgen deficiencies in women needs to consider *the hormonal singularity* of each woman. These future studies, on a large scale, will discuss the general framework of biology and the hormonal uniqueness of aging.

Warning

Mesterolone is not approved by the FDA and thus is not available in the United States; however, it is available worldwide. The misunderstanding about testosterone creates a lot of confusion. The FDA should quickly sponsor studies on the benefits of mesterolone in menopausal women. Any treatment needs the advice of a health-care professional. But first, doctors need to be aware of mesterolone treatment for androgen deficiency in women, after FDA approval.

At Which Age to Begin the Treatment?

Signs of sexual aging and general aging, caused by low levels of male hormones, are indications of the need for *precise and well-dosed* hormonal replacement treatment, which is necessary from the first symptoms. When those appear, hormonal insufficiency has already been in place for many months or many years. Early preventive therapy eliminates the most regressive phenomena. It is too late to act when there is significant sclerosis. Hormonal treatment can begin at any age to recover what can be and to avoid the aggravation of degeneration. The ideal would be a prevention of aging from the appearance of the first clinical symptom and even before. An annual clinical and biological checkup should be carried out systematically from age forty, or sooner, to prevent hormonal insufficiency in time.

Which Hormones to Take?

Androgens can be managed easily in women through percutaneous or oral delivery.

Percutaneous Delivery—Pellets

This method uses implantable testosterone pellets or cutaneous patches of testosterone. The FDA has approved neither of them.

Oral Method

This therapy is the easiest to handle. The leading hormone is mesterolone, available since 1966 worldwide, except for the United States and France.

> Mesterolone is a safe drug that has been around for over 50 years when it was used to treat male infertility. In 2019, a clinical discovery demonstrated that this molecule is a preventive treatment for diseases of aging in men and women [19].

Mesterolone is the best hormone for treating androgenic menopausal disease. It has the molecular characteristics of dihydrotestosterone, which is missing in the first stage of menopausal disease that initiates with sexual aging. Still, it also has molecular properties of testosterone, the levels of which also decrease during aging. Thus, it is possible to treat—on time and safely—the two stages of androgenic menopausal disease. The first stage is the pathological decrease in dihydrotestosterone production. The second stage is the pathological decrease of dihydrotestosterone and testosterone production.

Treatment consists of taking hormones in the form of sectile tablets of twenty-five milligrams labeled “for use in men only.” They are several types on the market. From those tablets, a compounding preparation is made by the pharmacist at lower doses appropriate for women, as prescribed by a medical professional. The maximum concentration of mesterolone in the blood is reached three hours after administration and then decreases until the eighth hour. The daily amount consists of two medication intakes: morning and middle of the day, or morning and evening.

The doses prescribed depend on the singularity of each woman. Mesterolone does not transform into the female hormone (estradiol—the dangerous proliferative hormone). At doses of five or ten milligrams, mesterolone prevents and cures urinary problems, pain during intercourse, and some diseases of aging in women. This topic was presented at the Spanish Society of Anti-Aging Medicine and Longevity (SEMAL) congress in Madrid in October 2015 [14].

Contraindications—Warning

Hormonal pharmaceuticals are accompanied by a note that gives specific explanations on the use of the drug. The formulation of contraindications is often brief. With any hormonal treatment imperatively having to be done under medical control, a specialized doctor will fix the necessary doses.

A lack of indication is the first contraindication. It is useless to take male hormones when the treatment is not necessary. The second contraindication is the incapacity of a woman to understand the effects of hormones. Finally, an inability to control food intake is a contraindication for hormonal replacement.

The future problems that come from androgenic menopausal disease can be prevented through treatment with mesterolone—a safe androgen mimetic. The dogma of estrogen and progesterone replacement after menopause is so entrenched in the mind-set of physicians that despite warnings from the FDA, one in two physicians still prescribes these "treatments." Mesterolone is used in men for decades and in women since 1998.

Renal, cardiac, and severe hepatic insufficiency cause serious disorders for which it is advisable to consider the hormonal effects. In those cases, we are, unfortunately, beyond prevention.

Harmful Side Effects

Excesses of weight, water, and salt retention are the consequences of a misconducted hormonal treatment in which overdosing occurs. These same phenomena are noted in women who take considerable and inadequate amounts of female hormones. The signs of overdose disappear after the suspension of excessive hormonal treatment. Reduced and adapted quantities are necessary to avoid the same perverse effects. The taking of male hormones increases protein synthesis. If, at the same time, food is in excess, overweight is inevitable. Treatment with male hormones requires the comprehension of their effects and a reflection on oneself, which imposes the control of nutrition. In the absence of consideration and planned effort, a woman treated with male hormones evolves in the same way that a calf treated with hormones does. The calf does not think. It eats. Thanks to anabolic hormones, it eats more. It then weighs more—to the greatest happiness of the lousy meat merchants. It is entirely possible to take hormones and lose weight with proper knowledge of nutrition.

Liver overload can occur when there is an overdose or incapacity to control food. However, there is a synthetic hormone that can be poorly tolerated by the liver: 17-alpha-methyl testosterone (available in the United States). Its use is dangerous. On the other hand, hepatic tolerance of mesterolone is remarkable.

When the hormonal balance is right, monitoring of the hormonal profile and maintenance treatment is done once a year. One monitors the function of the liver at the same time. Since the beginning of my clinical experience, I have not seen a single case of hepatic intolerance. On the contrary, some examples of hepatic insufficiency improved thanks to mesterolone treatment. It seems to have a regenerating effect on hepatic cells.

I have supervised permanently, with the assistance of many collaborators, thousands of patients following a hormonal replacement treatment with male hormones since 1974. I have never noted adverse effects caused by the correct administration of androgens, nor in their use in women since 1998.

Doping

Doping has occupied the pages of sporting magazines for many years. High-level sportswomen increase their muscular mass, and consequently their performance, by taking anabolic drugs, among which testosterone or its derivatives occupy a place of choice.

Young athletes generally have a normal secretion of male hormones. They do not, consequently, have any medical reason to take these drugs. They possess the advantage of having a natural output of male hormones higher than that of their elders, who are unable to win at the Olympic Games after age forty, their natural energy lacking male hormones over the years.

The challenges are considerable; individual young athletes do not hesitate to infringe on the sporting law and take anything that might enhance performance. Swallowing the tablets with frenzy, they are doped temporarily for transitory successes, endangering their health. Useless, awkward, and excessive absorption of hormones can cause all kinds of harmful side effects.

The public and even doctors then make an incorrect connection between doping problems and the therapeutic use of male hormones. With unreasoned fears, they say that hormones are harmful. Sex hormones are necessary for life. It is their perverse use that is harmful.

Treatment and Maintenance

Insulin is not prescribed blindly; it is the same with androgens.

Each woman is singular. Her biology varies during aging. Therefore, hormonal analyses are unique during life and according to the treatments. Treatment with hormones always needs the control of a doctor.

Overdose appears immediately through excessive nervousness. It is enough to reduce the amount gradually to find the proper quantity. The treatment continues with the daily taking of an optimal hormonal amount, twice a day.

The more surprising effect of mesterolone maintenance treatment is to prevent sexual aging and delay the general aging of the human body. It is a long-term effect, primarily preventive, which requires from the woman a reflection on herself. Treatment must continue throughout life.

Monitoring the Treatment

The amount of testosterone and dihydrotestosterone in the blood is already significant. If androgen metabolism is to be studied, the androgen pool should be analyzed. In all cases, under the control of a doctor, the following aspects of monitoring apply:

- Maintain your blood pressure, close to 12/8, and a pulse of 72 bpm.
- Avoid unreasonable weight gain (fat or muscle) by controlling food and exercise.
- Check your blood:
    - evolution of the number of red and white blood cells
    - glucose, urea, cholesterol, triglycerides (fats)
    - fluidity (antithrombin and other fluidity agents) and proteins
    - total bilirubin (liver indicator)

All these data help to determine the dose of mesterolone necessary to stabilize these parameters for overall improvement with time.

Is Long-Term Treatment with Androgens without Danger?

Since 1974, I have prescribed androgens in men, and I have prescribed mesterolone in women since 1998. I have never seen a pathological side effect. Among many doctors having followed this therapeutic method, according to my indications, none has ever told me of any incident in men or women. Well-proportioned hormonal treatment stabilizes the prostate (see *Ageless Man*). It is also useful in women with *androgenic disease of menopause* or bladder problems (chapter5).

It seems to me that the great caution of the FDA about HRT could be made yet more relevant by considering *androgenic disease of menopause*, and the need is urgent [14]. That is the real cause of most disorders after menopause. Biochemical and clinical studies could confirm this very quickly in a few months. In short, it is a question of measuring the metabolism of dihydrotestosterone in the blood and urine. The results will reveal the levels that are standard in women who have no problem before or after menopause. They will also show abnormal levels in women with insufficient production of dihydrotestosterone.

Treatment with a physiological dose of mesterolone eliminates disorders and normalizes biological levels. In case of doubt, just measure testosterone and dihydrotestosterone in the blood. If there is no pathological symptom, there is no disease. And if there is no disease, no treatment is necessary.

> Mesterolone replacement therapy will be of benefit to all those cases with persisting troubles due to decreased testosterone **and dihydrotestosterone** secretion.

Practical Matters

The Doctor

In an older general population of over age forty, any doctor is confronted each day with androgenic menopausal disease, particularly with its cardiovascular consequences, cerebral problems, and so on (see part III of this book). Consultation with the family doctor often concludes with the prescription of a cholesterol-lowering medication for cardiovascular disease, an anti-inflammatory drug for osteoarthritis, and antidepressant medication in the cases of depression. These traditional treatments are entirely justified. However, the results could be improved by treating the defective androgen hormone production.

The *well-proportioned* mesterolone treatment acts on all of the degraded structures. A biological study is necessary for each person. The appropriate amounts vary according to the constitution of each woman and modifications of her biology during the time of treatment.

Today, we are in the era of twenty-first-century medicine, computerized, scientific medicine. Biological results must be visualized in tables to understand the coordination of elements at a given time and to understand their evolution over time.

These data are explained in detail to the person being treated. Cooperation between the doctor and patient is essential. The patient will be able to take part by reviewing the table of results. The consultation lasts forty-five minutes to one hour. It takes place every three months until the moment when the coordinated hormonal biology is correct according to the data. Then control is done every six months. If everything is right, one visits the doctor once a year. Therapy is for life.

It takes at least ten years of practice to have experience in this kind of treatment. Indeed, the stabilized patient requires only ten specialized medical visits in ten years. However, the experience could be faster for the physician working in a dedicated center consulted by many patients. The ability to compare data with the use of computerized tables is significant and essential.

Male hormones are not aspirin. Androgenic menopausal disease, like any disease, requires medical treatment from the referring physician. Physicians will always seek the expert advice of an endocrinologist if needed.

Analyses

Hormonal measurement has been executed with precision since 1974 when reference laboratories developed radioimmunoassay methods. When a laboratory makes the analyses, it is preferable not to change them or take another laboratory's measurements because methods of analysis can differ from one laboratory to another. For each laboratory, it is necessary to remake the biological tables by considering the standards of this unique laboratory.

Drugs

The treatment for *androgenic menopausal disease* is mesterolone. Its formulation, marketed for more than twenty-five years, is no longer protected by a patent. Mesterolone is available worldwide, except for France and the United States. Doesn't androgenic menopausal disease exist in these countries?

Pharmaceutical Industry

We should wonder why pharmaceutical companies have no interest in marketing drugs that can prevent the diseases of aging? At the same time, the world market needs to sell cholesterol-lowering, antidiabetic, antihypertensive, antirheumatic, and antidepressive drugs. Human beings need those drugs for the moment because they have not been treated in the past to prevent diseases of aging. We are waiting for a leader in the pharmaceutical world who will quickly have a vision of the future and invest in getting manufactured anti-aging drugs on the market now, without delay. One of those existing drugs is mesterolone, whose anti-aging properties are unrecognized. The problem now is taking the first step in the right direction.

Medical Insurance

When anti-aging treatments are embraced, the services, performance, and profits of medical insurance companies will increase as a result of the availability of internet medical information. Insurers will be able to propose new insurance programs (e.g., life insurance) founded on scientific results that modify the mortality tables. Medical insurance and life insurance of the twenty-first century will consider medical departments specialized in the prevention of aging diseases, integrated into the medical structures of every nation.

Teaching

Today, one notes the interest of the new generation of doctors in the clinical and therapeutic concepts confirmed over the years in scientific publications. The teaching of the principles described in this book is not yet integrated into traditional university education. Many years, perhaps even many generations of teachers will be necessary before medical students and the medical community understand the pathology of androgenic menopausal disease, its causes, its consequences, and its treatment for the prevention of aging diseases. New teachers are necessary.

The Georges Debled, MD, Research Foundation has the aim of diffusing the teaching of the clinical and therapeutic principles of Dr. Georges Debled, not only to the medical community but also to women and men who want to understand the problems of aging. The website of the foundation, www.georgesdebled.org, updated continuously, makes it possible for all individuals to understand the aspects of their health problems concerning diseases of aging and particularly their initial causes. I have published or spoken about the principles exposed in this book in the medical press and the global media, in many congresses, on television networks, and the radio since 1974. The website of the foundation enumerates this work. It is an expression of a conceptual continuum into perpetual becoming.

Clinical and scientific research are essential components of anti-aging treatments. In clinical practice, the replacement of diseased cells with other cells, genetic corrections, and the substitution of anti-aging factors will always have to consider the pathology and treatment of *androgenic menopausal disease.*

A Tsunami of Aging Diseases

We can see the arrival of a tsunami of aging diseases. Among these diseases, dementia occupies a worrying place. With the graying of the world's population, the projections of the World Health Organization (WHO) predict that the number of people who have dementia will triple from the current 50 million to reach 82 million in 2030 and 152 million by 2050.

Because the diseases of aging develop over forty years and lead to death, we can predict that in 2060, we will witness the extinction of a particular population made up of those women and men who did not receive preventive treatment for diseases of aging.

The annual cost of dementia worldwide is approximately $818 billion. By 2030, this cost will more than double to $2 trillion.

There are currently ten million new cases of dementia per year because the prevention of this disease of aging is not yet standard practice.

Anti-aging therapy includes the treatment of androgenic diseases of menopause and andropause [14–17]. This treatment may prevent, among other things, the development of arteriosclerosis, which is responsible for the highest number of dementia cases [18–19].

Treatment for androgenic diseases of menopause and andropause is now available. The results are more effective with controlled nutrition. By the time the tsunami of diseases of aging hits, it will be too late.

HMS WORLD

Prevention of aging diseases is relevant to the medicine of the twenty-first century. The company HMS WORLD manages the Georges Debled, MD, Research Foundation that is dedicated to research on aging diseases.

HMS WORLD is also a consultant company that will help doctors and their patients to manage anti-aging treatments.

www.hmsworld.net

www.georgesdebled.org

Thank you for your interest.

If you have comments or questions, please send an email to

contact@hmsworld.net

Conclusion

Ageless Woman

By the knowledge of hormones,
are we not the day before to get
the hand on the development of our
body—and of the brain itself?

—Teilhard de Chardin,
The Human Phenomenon

Grow Young Again: How to Cure and Prevent Diseases of Aging

Since the end of the seventeenth century, times have not changed much for humans. Yes, one notes a progressive lengthening of longevity, and one speaks about a fourth or even a fifth and sixth age. This remarkable phenomenon is the result of the fulgurating progress of medicine for about fifty years, from a time when one lived, on average, twenty years less than today.

Androgenic menopausal disease and senility provoke devastation that puts health-care systems in danger.

The untreated androgenic menopausal disease causes a progressive reduction in sexual capacities and starts the vicious cycle of self-destruction, leading to death. Considerable sums are necessary today to fight against the diseases of aging. But medical technology seems condemned to save fewer and fewer patients by neglecting the prevention of their organs' degeneration.

The traditional conception of cardiovascular disease is unaware of the essential principle of vital energy sources. The years that precede cardiac arrest or the fatal arterial thrombosis are, in general, lived with multiple and dramatic incidents. The economic and social costs of cardiovascular disease are gigantic, comprising the most significant financial balance of the health-care economy. Degenerative cardiovascular diseases are never cured. They are looked after and operated on, but patients have relapses and worsen unrelentingly.

The cardiac patient depends more and more on medical technology. Cardiac transplants are spectacular but don't last. The new heart grafted in a woman with androgenic menopausal disease degenerates with the receiver's body, with the coronary arteries obstructing it quickly. How is it that traditional therapy for cardiovascular disease does not consider the energy sources necessary for the contractions of the musculature, heart, and arteries? Glycogen and contractile proteins constitute the energy needed for the arterial and cardiac muscle to function, thanks to male hormones. Degeneration of the heart and blood vessels is a consequence of the lack of energetic factors. In their absence, the contraction of the heart weakens, the arteries narrow, and the veins become varicose. Even if an artificial heart replaces the diseased heart, the whole of the body degenerates.

A lack of energetic factors acts directly on the composition of the blood: the number of red blood cells falls, the cholesterol levels and blood sugar rise, and the blood fluidity (antithrombin III) drops. A woman with *androgenic menopausal disease* has a weak heart that propels her fatty and viscous blood through narrowed arteries. She takes all kinds of drugs to regulate her heart, reduce her hypertension, thin her blood, and lower her sugar and cholesterol levels. All of those functions can be carried out naturally by male hormones.

The excess weight of the population continues to increase overall and regularly, causing an increasingly high death rate due to ignorance of food guidelines. Certain women, conscious of their excess of weight, make desperate efforts to find a standard silhouette, increasingly necessary in a society that eliminates those who do not impress. The many slimming regimes are complicated to follow because they do not consider the role of male hormones in regulating the metabolism of fat and sugar. In a perpetually unbalanced state, some individuals abandon diets as a rule. Thus, they end up resembling a fatty grandmother without being able to hope to live longer than she did.

Eye and hearing troubles, widespread after age fifty, are closely related to the degeneration of sense organs; one can no longer be unaware of the role of male hormones in their integrity and structure.

By 1998, I had described the mechanisms of genital aging in women (chapters 5–7). Preventive medication with mesterolone makes it possible to preserve sexual function, at the same time avoiding urinary problems.

Osteoarthritis is an infirmity of senescence. It is invalidating and painful, and its medical and social costs burden health-care budgets to excess. Orthopedic surgery repairs the joint articulations of older and disabled women. Prostheses can replace practically all joints. Individuals are even assisted today by successive and perilous replacements of hip prostheses. The damage is often severe, and patients are often uneasy about reparative surgery.

Care of arthroses requires a real industry. It implements battalions of doctors and medical staff members, although it is true that the treatment of symptoms never cures osteoarthritis.

Osseous brittleness and degeneration are closely related to a lack of male hormones. In their absence, patients will experience new articular blockings and other fractures in a process that will not end.

Lastly, depression and melancholy in certain women with *androgenic menopausal disease* are frequent and lead to their retirement around age sixty. Their brains, deprived of male hormones, are unable to face the requirements of an external world. Ousted from social and economic structures, they do not have any future, whereas their human and professional resources could be useful if they were to recover their vital energy.

Metamorphosis and Rebirth of Women beyond Age Forty

Formerly, as a result of ignorance, fatalism accepted the diseases of aging—one aged without hope of better days. Reduction in sexual activity inevitably led to a lack of libido. One did not speak about it. Death was premature. Things were just so.

Many women still think they are not able to change any aspects of their aging, mainly due to a lack of information.

Since the end of the Second World War, scientific knowledge has made extraordinary progress. Computers exceed the capacities of the human brain. Researchers handle genes with the hope of eliminating genetic diseases. In short, all seems possible.

During this time, however, women age badly and degenerate in the millions, endangering the balance of societies. This phenomenon is paradoxical and completely anachronistic according to current knowledge. Certain women are conscious of that. Suffering from menopausal troubles, whereas all was well a few months before, they cannot accept the idea that medical science cannot cure them; they have questioned this a hundred times. While wanting to live in good health, they do not ask for anything more than a life supplement.

It is necessary to reactivate their biological program, which arrived at the end of its average duration.

The fundamental mistake is to consider that it is possible to delay the aging of women by administering female hormones, which are not necessary after menopause.

Replacement of the missing male hormones restarts sexual activity but also prolongs the biological mechanisms of life. Good sexual activity and the absence of menopausal troubles reflect good health.

The general degradations appear around age forty, with a moderate rise in blood pressure, some excess weight, craving for sugars, an increase in blood cholesterol, small cardiac alarms, and stiffness of movement. Very often, the silhouette has already changed. This is a sign that does not mislead.

Male hormones act on the various structures of the organism. Sharp observers understand that health concerns the whole of the body. Is there hope? Undoubtedly. The metamorphosis is possible. Women with menopausal disease can change, just as the caterpillar becomes the chrysalis.

For that to occur, the second surprise is that she must increase her consciousness and acquire more soul. To take hormones to live longer without better living is entirely contradictory. Vital efforts are necessary to understand and implement rigorous control of food, harmonious physical exercise, oxygenation, and relaxation. This program, however simple, often goes against monolithic habits. After reflection, change happens little by little.

The third surprise is the complete metamorphosis at the end of the road. The regenerated woman, in full possession of her mental faculties, can finally release herself from material contingencies, a requirement of true rebirth. The chrysalis becomes a butterfly.

Ageless Woman

The treatment and prevention of diseases of aging will have a considerable effect on the social, economic, and cultural fields because the life cycle of the human being will change.

Today, the regressive woman can only truly realize herself for between twenty and forty years. She then regresses unrelentingly up to eighty years. The times of the backward woman are now the times of the ageless woman.

With knowledge and the use of hormones, today's women can prevent sexual aging, which precedes senile involution and its many diseases. She can see herself in twenty years—she will no longer suffer from the androgenic disease of menopause, senescence, and decline. "Just be" will be her reason to live.

The ageless woman lives a continued revitalization. One cannot estimate her longevity.

We are still unaware of where the long-term treatment of sexual aging and other biological aging will lead. We will eventually combine treatments involving cell regeneration with the knowledge of nucleic acids and cell "mothers" that condition cellular division.

Genetic research has made significant progress. Soon, it will complement the dynamic biochemistry of the human body, and what is already known about *androgenic disease of menopause and andropause.*

From this time on, a formidable race begins to control one's lifetime. The future of women is closely related to knowledge of the biological mechanisms of the female body, as described in this book. The digitalization of all physiological parameters of each person must be the standard.

The prevention of diseases of aging is already possible. Revitalization with mesterolone after age forty is necessary to avoid the decline. Other biological deficiencies that should appear later will be considered. This is the future principal activity for new medical professionals. Attempting to correct Alzheimer's disease at seventy years of age is almost impossible. It is at age forty that research and prevention must begin.

Regressive Woman	**Ageless Woman**
Birth	Birth
Childhood	Childhood
Adolescence	Adolescence
Adulthood	
Androgenic Menopausal Disease	Menopause
Senescence	Adulthood
Senility	
Death	?

The ageless woman is already born. Do you want to be her? Think and act now.

July 24, 2020

Bibliography

1

Sexual and Reproductive Aging Announces Degeneration of All Structures of the Female Body

1.BAULIEU E-E. AND KELLY PAUL A. Hormones. Hermann publishers,1990.

2. DEBLED G. The menopausal disease. Approaches to aging control: 19:17-24, October 2015.

3. ZUMOFF B, STRAIN GW, MILLER LK, ROSNER W. Twenty-four hours mean plasma testosterone concentration decline with age in normal premenopausal women. J Clin Endocrinol Metab, 1995, 80:1429-1430.

4. FOGLE RH1, STANCZYK FZ, ZHANG X, PAULSON RJ. Ovarian androgen production in postmenopausal women. J Clin Endocrinol Metab. 2007 Aug;92(8):3040-3. Epub 2007 May 22.

5. ROSSOUW JE, ANDERSON GL, PRENTICE RL, LACROIX AZ, KOOPERBERG C, et al. Risks and benefits of estrogen plus progestin in healthy postmenopausal women: principal results From the Women's Health Initiative randomized controlled trial. JAMA. 2002; 288:321–333.

2

Male Hormones, Keys to Menopause Troubles

1. ROBEL P. -Mode d'Action des Androgènes : Les Androgènes. Rapports présentés à la XVe réunion des endocrinologistes de langue française : 20-38. Athènes, 6-8 septembre 1979. -MASSON PARIS NEW YORK BARCELONE MILAN 1979.

2. MICHEL G., BAULIEU E.E., et COURRIER R. -Récepteur Cytosoluble des Androgènes dans un Muscle Strié Squelettique : C.R. Acad. Sc. Paris, 279 : 421-424, 1974.

3. BLASIUS R., KAFER K., SEITZ W. - Untersuchungen über die Wirkung von Testosteron auf die Kontraktilen Strukturproteine des Herzens. Klin. Woch., 34, 11/12, 324, 1956.

4. AL MADHOUN AS, VORONOVA A, RYAN T, ZAKARIYAH A, MCINTIRE C, GIBSON L, SHELTON M, RUEL M, SKERJANC IS. Testosterone enhances cardiomyogenesis in stem cells and recruits the Androgen Receptor to the MEF2C and HCN4 genes. J Mol Cell Cardiol. 2013 Apr 15. Elsevier Ltd.

5. CONSTANTINE A. STRATAKIS AND NEAL S. YOUNG, RODRIGO T. CALADO, WILLIAM T. YEWDELL, KEISHA L. WILKERSON, JOSHUA A. REGAL, SACHIKO KAJIGAYA. Sex hormones, acting on the TERT gene, increase telomerase activity in human primary hematopoietic cells. Blood journal. Hematology library.org by guest on October 22, 2012.

6. GUAY A MUNARRIZ R, JACOBSON J, TALAKOUB L, TRAISH A, QUIRK F. GOLDSTEIN I, SPARK R. Serum androgen levels in healthy premenopausal women with and without sexual dysfunction: Part A. Serum androgen levels in women aged 20-49 years with no complaints of sexual dysfunction. International Journal of Impotence Research, 2004, 16:112-120.

7. GUAY A JACOBSON J, MUNANIZ R, TRAISH A. TALAKOUB L, QUIRK F, GOLDSTEIN I, SPARK R. PART B: reduced serum androgen levels in healthy premenopausal women with complaints of sexual dysfunction. International Journal of Impotence Research, 2004. 16:121-129

3.

Treatment with Male Hormones Is an Old Concept

1. BUTENANDT A. & K TSCHERNING, « Über Androsteron, ein Krystallisiertes Männliches Sexualhormon. I Isolierung und Reindarstellung aus Männerharn », *Z. Physiol. Chem. Bd.*, n° 229, 1934, p. 167–184.

2. SHORR E, PAPANICOLAOU GN, STIMMEL BF. Neutralization of ovarian follicular hormone in women by simultaneous administration of male sex hormone. Proc Soc Exp Bio Med 1938; 38:759-62.

3. LOESER AA. The action of testosterone propionate on the uterus and breast. Lancet 1938; 1:373-4.

4. BERLIND M. Oral administration of methyltestosterone in gynecology. J Clin Endocrinol 1941; 1:986-91.

5. SALMON UJ. Rational for androgen therapy in gynecology. J Clin Endocrinol 1941; 1:162-79.

6. BRUCHOVSKY N. and WILSON J.D., The Conversion of Testosterone to 5α-Androstan-17β-ol-3-one by Rat Prostate in Vivo and in Vitro. The Journal of Biological Chemistry. Vol. 243, № 8, Issue of April 25, pp2012-2021, 1968

7. ANDERSON K.M. and SHUTSUNG LIAO, Selective Retention of Dihydrotestosterone by Prostatic Nuclei. Nature 219, 277-279 (20 July 1968)

8. Society of Obstetricians and Gynaecologists of Canada: Canadian Consensus Conference on Menopause, 2006 Update. J Obstet. Gynaecol. Can 2006 ;28(2 Suppl 1): S7-S94.

9. DEBLED G.- L'Andropause, cause, conséquences et remèdes. Maloine, Paris, 1988.

10. DEBLED G. Andropause. 1 : Le castrat : un modèle "expérimental". N° 4308 - 24 mai 1989. Le Quotidien du Médecin. Paris.

11. DEBLED G. Andropause 2 : Dépister pour reculer le vieillissement prématuré. N° 43 l 3 - 3 l mai 1989. Le Quotidien du Médecin. Paris.

12. DEBLED G. Andropause 3 : Sclérose des corps caverneux : le fatalisme n'est plus de mise. N° 4318 - 7 juin 1989. Le Quotidien du Médecin. Paris.

13. DEBLED G. Andropause 4 : Les troubles "émotionnels" ne doivent pas cacher l'impuissance organique. N° 4323 - 14 juin 1989. Le Quotidien du Médecin. Paris.

14. DEBLED G. Andropause 5 : Les troubles de l'éjaculation. N° 4328 - 21 juin 1989. Le Quotidien du Médecin. Paris.

15. DEBLED G. Andropause 6 : Les perturbations de la miction. N° 4334 - 29 juin 1989. Le Quotidien du Médecin. Paris.

16. DEBLED G. Andropause 7 : L'atrophie de la prostate. N° 4372 - 26 septembre 1989. Le Quotidien du Médecin. Paris. Le Quotidien du Médecin. Paris.

17. DEBLED G. Andropause 8 : Des difficultés mictionnelles à l'insuffisance rénale. N° 4377 - 3 octobre 1989. Le Quotidien du Médecin. Paris.

18. DEBLED G. Andropause 9 : Un âge où "tout se dégrade". N° 4382 - 10 octobre 1989. Le Quotidien du Médecin. Paris.

19. DEBLED G. Andropause 10 : Les hormones sexuelles de l'homme. N4337 - 17 octobre l 989. Le Quotidien du Médecin. Paris.

20. DEBLED G. Andropause 11 : Le généraliste et l'exploration du vieillissement sexuel. N° 4397 - 31 octobre 1989. Le Quotidien du Médecin. Paris.

21. DEBLED G. Andropause 12 : Les androgènes favorisent-ils l'apparition d'un cancer de la prostate ? N° 4401 - 7 novembre 1989. Le Quotidien du Médecin. Paris.

22. DEBLED G. Andropause 13 : Le traitement hormonal. N° 4422 - 6 décembre 1989. Le Quotidien du Médecin. Paris.

23. DEBLED G. Au-delà de celle limite votre ticket est toujours valables. Albin Michel. 1992.Paris.

24. DEBLED G. The male climacteric, prime cause of sex involution. The Tenth annual international symposium on man and his environment in health and disease. February 27-March 1, 1992. Dallas. Texas. The U.S.A.

25. DEBLED G. The male climacteric, prime cause of aging. The Tenth annual international symposium on man and his environment in health and disease. February 27-March 1, 1992. Dallas. Texas. The U.S.A.

26. DEBLED G. Le traitement hormonal du vieillissement sexuel de l'homme. Journal de médecine esthétique et de chirurgie dermatologique. Vol XXII-N° 85: 7 - 16, 1995

27. DEBLED G. La enfermedad "andropausia". Congreso internacional de medicina anti envejecimiento. Septiembre 21-22 y 23 de 2006 Club Militar de Bogotá. Bogotá D.C.

28. DEBLED G. Atrofia de la próstata y envejecimiento. Congreso internacional de medicina anti envejecimiento. Septiembre 21-22 y 23 de 2006 Club Militar de Bogotá. Bogotá D.C.

29. DEBLED G. La enfermedad "andropausia". Mi experiencia hace 32 años. International congress of anti-aging Medicine Vº congreso de la sociedad española de medicina anti envejecimiento y longevidad. Madrid 3,4 y 5 de noviembre 2006. Hotel Melia Castilla. Madrid.

30. DEBLED G. The menopausal disease.
Approaches to aging control: 19:17-24, October 2015.

31. DEBLED G. Ageless Man. HMS Editions. 2017

32. DEBLED G. The androgenic disease of andropause. SEMAL congress, Seville. October 5, 2019.

5

Aging of Women's Masculine Genitalia

1. BAULIEU E-E. AND KELLY PAUL A. Hormones. Hermann publishers,1990.

2. ZUMOFF B, STRAIN GW, MILLER LK, ROSNER W. Twenty-four hours mean plasma testosterone concentration decline in non-premenopausal women. J Clin Endocrinol Metab, 1995, 80:1429-1430.

3. MASSAFRA C, DE FELICE C, AGNUSDEI DP, GIOIA D, BAGNOLI F. Department of Obstetrics and Gynecology, University of Siena, Italy. Androgens and osteocalcin during the menstrual cycle. J Clin Endocrinol Metab. 1999 Mar;84(3):971-4.

4. DEBLED G. The menopausal disease. Approaches to aging control : 19:17-24, October 2015.

5. DEBLED G. -La Pathologie obstructive Congénitale de l'Uretère Terminal. Thèse d'agrégation de l'enseignement supérieur en Sciences Urologiques, Université Libre de Bruxelles, 18 Mai 1971 : Acta Urol. Belg., 39 : 371-465, 1971.

6. BALDASSARRE M1, PERRONE AM, GIANNONE FA, ARMILLOTTA F, BATTAGLIA C, COSTANTINO A, VENTUROLI S, MERIGGIOLA MC. Androgen receptor expression in the human vagina under different physiological and treatment conditions. Int J Impot Res. 2013 Jan;25(1):7-11.

6

Aging of the Reproductive Organs

1. LEE JENNIFER S 1, BRUCE ETTINGER, FRANK Z STANCZYK, ERIC VITTINGHOFF, VLADIMIR HANES, JANE A CAULEY, WALT CHANDLER, JIM SETTLAGE, MARY S BEATTIE, ELIZABETH FOLKERD, MITCH DOWSETT, DEBORAH GRADY, STEVEN R CUMMINGS. Comparison of Methods to Measure Low Serum Estradiol Levels in Postmenopausal Women. J Clin Endocrinol Metab. 2006 Oct;91(10):3791-7.

2. DAVID J. PORTMAN, MD, MARGERY L.S. GASS, MD, NCMP, on behalf of the vulvovaginal atrophy terminology consensus conference panel. Genitourinary syndrome of menopause: new terminology for vulvovaginal atrophy from the International Society for the Study of Women's Sexual Health and The North American Menopause Society. Menopause: The Journal of The North American Menopause Society Vol. 21, No. 10, pp. 1063/1068, 2014.

3. DEBLED G. The menopausal disease. Approaches to aging control: 19:17-24, October 2015.

7

Premature Genital Aging

1. DEBLED G. Mesterolone pharmaceutical composition for dihydrotestosterone deficiencies in the woman. EP 2687215 B1.

2. HARRISON'S principes de médicine interne. Conséquences des troubles contraceptifs oraux avec une diminution de la synthèse des androgènes de l'ovaire–331 : Maladies de l'ovaire et de l'appareil génital féminin : p. 1832-1833, 1988.

3. ISAKSSON E, VON SCHOULTZ E, ODLIND V, SODERQVIST G, CSEMICZKY G, CARLSTROM K, SKOOG L, VON SCHOULTZ B. Effects of oral contraceptives on breast epithelial proliferation. Cancer Res Treat 2001 Jan; 65(2):163-169

4. KAHLENBORN C, MODUGNO F, POTTER DM, SEVERS WB. Oral contraceptive use as a risk factor for premenopausal breast cancer: a meta-analysis. Mayo Clin Proc. 2006 Oct;81(10):1290-302.

5. CHRISTOPHER I. LI, ELISABETH F. BEABER, MEI TZU CHEN TANG, PEGGY L. PORTER, JANET R. DALING, KATHLEEN E. MALONE Effect of Depo-Medroxyprogesterone Acetate on Breast Cancer Risk among Women 20 to 44 Years of Age. Cancer Res; 72(8); 2028–35.2012

6. CHLEBOWSKI RT1, HENDRIX SL, LANGER RD, STEFANICK ML, GASS M, LANE D, RODABOUGH RJ, GILLIGAN MA, CYR MG, THOMSON CA, KHANDEKAR J, PETROVITCH H, MCTIERNAN A; WHI Investigators. Influence of estrogen plus progestin on breast cancer and mammography in healthy postmenopausal women: The Women's Health Initiative Randomized Trial. JAMA. 2003 Jun 25;289(24):3243-53.

7. PANZER *and al.* Impact of Oral Contraceptives on Sex hormone-binding Globulin and Androgen Levels: A Retrospective Study in Women with Sexual Dysfunction. The Journal of Sexual Medicine, January 2006;3: p.104-113

8. COELINGH BENNINK H. J. T., HOLINKA C. F. and DICZFALUSY E. Estetrol review: profile and potential clinical applications. CLIMACTERIC 2008; II (Suppl 1):47-58.

9. HERJAN J.T. COELINGH BENNINK, MD, Ph.D., CAROLE VERHOEVEN, Ph.D., YVETTE ZIMMERMAN, Ph.D., MONIQUE VISSER, Ph.D., JEAN-MICHEL FOIDART, MD, Ph.D., AND KRISTINA GEMZELL-DANIELSSON, MD, Ph.D. Pharmacodynamic effects of the fetal estrogen estetrol in postmenopausal women: results from a multiple-rising-dose study. Menopause: The Journal of The North American Menopause Society. Vol. 24, No. 6, pp. 677-685, 2017.

10. BAULIEU E-E. AND KELLY PAUL A. Hormones. Hermann publishers,1990.

11. MASSAFRA C, DE FELICE C, AGNUSDEI DP, GIOIA D, BAGNOLI F. Department of Obstetrics and Gynecology, University of Siena, Italy. Androgens and osteocalcin during the menstrual cycle. J Clin Endocrinol Metab. 1999 Mar;84(3):971-4.

12. CANADIAN SOCIETY OF GYNAECOLOGISTS AND OBSTETRICIANS: Consensus Guideline on Continuous and Extended Hormonal Contraception. JOGC. Volume 29, Number 7. Supplement 2. July 2007.

13. Y. ZIMMERMANN M.J.C. EIJKEMANS, H.J.T. COELINGH BENNINK I, M.A. BLANKENSTEINT AND B.C.J.M. FAUSER. The effect of combined oral contraception on testosterone levels in healthy women: a systematic review and meta-analysis. Human Reproduction Update, Vo1.20, No.1 pp. 76-105, 2014

14. SHUSTER, LYNNE T.; RHODES, DEBORAH J.; GOSTOUT, BOBBIE S.; GROSSARDT, BRANDON R.; ROCCA, WALTER A. (2010). "Premature menopause or early menopause: Long-term health consequences." Maturitas. 2010, 65 (2) : 161-166

15. ROSSOUW JE, ANDERSON GL, PRENTICE RL, LACROIX AZ, KOOPERBERG C, et al. Risks and benefits of estrogen plus progestin in healthy postmenopausal women: principal results From the Women's Health Initiative randomized controlled trial. JAMA. 2002 ; 288:321-333.

16. DEBLED G. Composition pharmaceutique pour la contraception chez la femme. OPRI: 100072467. №2019/5904. 13 décembre 2019

8

Diabetes and Androgenic Menopausal Disease: The Sugar Mechanism

1, CATHERINE KIM, M.D., M.P.H. AND JEFFREY B. HALTER, M.D. Endogenous Sex Hormones, Metabolic Syndrome, and Diabetes in Men and Women. Curr Cardiol Rep. 2014 Apr; 16(4): 467.

2. WORLD HEALTH ORGANIZATION. Global health risks. Mortality and burden of disease attributable to selected significant risks. Geneva, 2009.

3. PELLEGRINI G. -L'Azione Antidiabetica degli Ormoni Sessuali Maschili nel quadro della Fisiopatologia del Diabete: Minerva Medica, 27: 1-9, 1947.

4. DOMINIQUE SIMON, MD, Ph.D., MARIE-ALINE CHARLES, MD, NAJIBA LAHLOU, MD, KHALIL NAHOUL, MD, JEAN-MICHEL OPPERT, MD, Ph.D., MICHE` LE GOUAULT-HEILMANN, MD, NICOLE LEMORT, BSC, NADINE THIBULT, BSC, EVELYNE JOUBERT, MD, BEVERLEY BALKAU, Ph.D., EVELINE ESCHWEGE, MD: Androgen Therapy Improves Insulin Sensitivity and Decreases Leptin Level in Healthy Adult Men With Low Plasma Total Testosterone. Diabetes care, volume 24, number 12, 2149-2151, December 2001

9

Male Hormones Against Cholesterol

1. LIPID RESEARCH PROGRAM -The Lipid Research Clinics Population Studies Data Book -NIH Publication No 80: 1527, vol 1 BETHESDA, 1980.

2. DAI W.S., MD, DrPH, GUTAI J.P., MD, KULLER L.H., MD, DrPH, LAPORTE R.E., PhD., FALVO-GERARD L., MPH, and GAGGIULA A., Ph.D. - Relation

between Plasma High-Density Lipoprotein Cholesterol and Sex Hormone Concentrations in Men: Am. J. Cardiol., 53: 1259-1263, 1984.

3. GUTAI J., LAPORTE R., KULLER J., DAI W., FALVO-GERARD L., CAGGIULA A. -Plasma Testosterone, High-Density Lipoprotein Cholesterol and other Lipoprotein Fractions: Am. J. Cardiol., 48: 897-902, 1981.

4. HOFMAN A, OTT A, BRETELER MM, BOTS ML, SLOOTER AJ, VAN HARSKAMP F, VAN DUIJN CN, VAN BROECKHOVEN C, GROBBEE DE.-Atherosclerosis, apolipoprotein E, and prevalence of dementia and Alzheimer's disease in the Rotterdam Study. Lancet. 1997 Jan 18;349(9046):151-4.

10

Excess Weight and Obesity: The Ideal Weight

1. LEW E.A. and GARFINKEL L. -Variations in Mortality by Weight among 750.000 Men and Women -J. Chron. Dis., 32: 563, 1979.

2. ZUMOFF B., STRAIN G.W., MILLER L.K., ROSNER W., SENIE R., SERES D.S., and ROSENFELD R.S. -Plasma Free and Non-Sex-Binding-Globulin-Bound Testosterone Are Decreased in Obese Men in Proportion to their Degree of Obesity: J. Clin. Endocrinol. Metabol., 71,4: 929-931, 1990.

11

Muscular Weakness

1. FORSTER D.W. - Diabète Sucré, 327 : 1778 dans HARRISON T.R.- Principes de Médecine Interne Médecine-Sciences Flammarion, Paris 1989.

2. BOREL J-P., RANDOUX A., MAQUARTF-X., LE PEUCH C., VALEYRE J.-Biochimie Dynamique -1421 : 1400. MALOINE DECARIE PARIS MONTREAL 1987.

3. JUNG I. and BEAULIEU E-E. -Testosterone Cytosol Receptor in the Rat Levator Ani Muscle: Nature New Biology, 237: 24-26, 1972.

4. GILLESPIE C.A. and EDGERTON V.R. -The role of Testosterone in Exercise-induced Glycogen Supercompensation: Horm. Metab. Res., 2: 364-366, 1970.

5. SERRA C, TANGHERLINI F, RUDY S, LEE D, TORALDO G, SANDOR NL, ZHANG A, JASUJA R, BHASIN S. Testosterone improves the regeneration of old and young mouse skeletal muscle. J Gerontol A Biol Sci Med Sci. 2013 Jan; 68(1):17-26.

6. RARIY CM, RATCLIFFE SJ, WEINSTEIN R, BHASIN S, BLACKMAN MR, CAULEY JA, ROBBINS J, ZMUDA JM, HARRIS TB, CAPPOLA AR. Higher serum free testosterone concentration in older women is associated with greater bone mineral density, lean body mass, and total fat mass: the cardiovascular health study. J Clin Endocrinol Metab. 2011 Apr;96(4):989-96. Epub 2011 Feb 2.

7. GORDON I. SMITH, JUN YOSHINO, DOMINIC N. REEDS, DAVID BRADLEY, RACHEL E. BURROWS, HENRY D. HEISEY, ANNA C. MOSELEY, AND BETTINA MITTENDORFER. Testosterone and Progesterone, But Not Estradiol, Stimulate Muscle Protein Synthesis in Postmenopausal Women. J Clin Endocrinol Metab. 2014 Jan; 99(1) : 256–265.12

12

Arteriosclerosis or Arterial Rigidity

1. National Centre for Health Statistics -Vital Statistics Report, Final Mortality Statistics, 1982.

2. BEST and TAYLOR - -Physiological Basis of Medical Practice: 155 WILLIAMS and WILKINS COMPAGNY BALTIMORE 1950.

3. DEBLED G. -La Pathologie obstructive Congénitale de l'Uretère Terminal -Thèse d'agrégation de l'enseignement supérieur en Sciences Urologiques, Université Libre de Bruxelles, 18 Mai 1971 : Acta Urol. Belg., 39 : 371-465, 1971.

4. GREGOIR W. et DEBLED G. -Méga-Uretère Congénital : Encyclopédie Médico-Chirurgicale, 18, Rue SEGUIER. PARIS VI 18158 E10 : 4-14 1971.

5. DEBLED G. -L'anatomie pathologique de l'uretère dilaté. Procès-verbaux, mémoires et discussions de l'Association Française d'Urologie, 67ème Session : 521-525, 1974.

6. DEBLED G. Hormone stéroïde pour la prévention de maladies associées au vieillissement. OPRI: 100072468. № 2019/5905. 13 décembre 2019.

13

Anemia

1. STEINGLASS P., GORDON A.S., CHARIPPER H.A. -Effect of Castration and Sex Hormones on Blood of the Rat: Proc. Soc. exp. Biol. Med., 48: 169-177, 1941.

2. KENNEDY B.J. and GILBERTSEN A.S. - Increased Erythropoiesis Induced by Androgenic Hormones: J. Clin. Invest. 35: 717, 1956.

3. KENNEDY B.J. - Fluoxymesterone in Advanced Breast Cancer: New Engl. J. Med., 259: 673, 1958.

4. SHAHIDI N.T. - Androgens and Erythropoiesis: N. Engl. J. Med., 289: 72-80, 1973.

5. NAJEAN Y. and coll. -Long Term Follow-up in Patients with Aplastic Anemia. A study of 137 Androgen-Treated Patients surviving more than Two Years: Am. J. Med., 71: 543-551, 1981.

6. CLAUSTRES M., BELLET H., SULTAN C.-Action des Androgènes sur les Cellules-Souches Erythroïdes en Culture : Ann. Biol. clin., 44 : 5-13, 1986.

7. LUIGI FERRUCCI, MARCELLO MAGGIO, STEFANIA BANDINELLI, SHEHZAD BASARIA, FULVIO LAURETANI, ALESSANDRO BLE, GIORGIO VALENTI, WILLIAM B. ERSHLER, JACK M. GURALNIK,, and DAN L. LONGO. Low

Testosterone Levels and the Risk of Anemia in Older Men and Women. Arch Intern Med. 2006 July 10; 166(13): 1380–1388.

14

Viscous Blood, Thromboses, Embolisms, Varicose Veins and Hemorrhoids

1. BONITHON-KOPP C., SCARABIN P.-Y., BARA L., CASTANIER M., JACQUESON A., and ROGER M. -Relationship between Sex Hormones and Haemostatic Factors in Healthy Middle-Aged Men: Atherosclerosis, 71: 71-76, 1988.

2. CARON Ph., SIE P., BENNET A., CAMARE R., BONEU B. et LOUVET J.P. -Testosterone Plasmatique et Inhibiteur Anti Activateur Tissulaire du Plasminogène Chez l'Homme : Ann. Endocrinol., 49, 6: 117C (182), 1988-8ème Congrès Français d'Endocrinologie, Bruxelles 3-5 Octobre 1988.

3. FEARNLEY G.R. and CHAKRABARTI R. -Increase of Blood Fibrinolytic Activity by Testosterone: The Lancet, July 21: 128-132, 1962.

4. WALKER I.D. and DAVIDSON J.F. -Long-Trem Fibrinolytic Enhancement with Anabolic Steroid Therapy: A Five Year Study: Progress in Chemical Fibrinolysis and Thrombosis, Vol 3: 491-499. Edited by J.F. DAVIDSON, R.M. ROWAN, M.M. SAMAMA, and P.C. DESNOYERS- RAVEN PRESS NEW YORK 1978.

5. WORLD HEALTH ORGANIZATION -Prevention of Ischaemic Heart Disease. Metabolic Aspects: WHO Symposium, WHO/CVD/73:3, MADRID1972.

6. SVETLANA KALINCHENKO, ALEXANDR ZEMLYANOY, AND LOUIS GOOREN. Improvement of the diabetic foot upon testosterone administration to hypogonadal men with peripheral arterial disease. Report of three cases. Cardiovascular Diabetology, 8: 19, 2009.

7. WIMAN B., LJUNGBERG B., CHMELIEWSKA J., URDEN G., BLOMBACK M. and JOHNSON H. -The Role of the Fibrinolitic System in Deep Vein Thrombosis: J. Lab. Clin. Med., 105: 265-270, 1985.

8. BROWSE N.L. and BURNAND K.G. -The Cause of Venous Ulceration: Lancet, II: 243-245, 1982.

9. BENNET A., CARON Ph., SIE P., LOUVET J.-P., et BAZEX J. -Ulcères de Jambe Post-Phlébitiques et Caryotype XYY : Tests de Fibrinolyse et Fonction Androgénique : Ann. Dermatol. Venereol., 114: 1097-1101, 1987.

15

Hypertension, Disease of the World

1. MERAI R, SIEGEL C, RAKOTZ M, BASCH P, WRIGHT J, WONG B; DHSC, THORPE P. CDC Grand Rounds: A Public Health Approach to Detect and Control Hypertension. MMWR Morb Mortal Wkly Rep. 2016 Nov 18;65(45):1261-1264.

2. BEST and TAYLOR - -Physiological Basis of Medical Practice: 155 WILLIAMS and WILKINS COMPANY BALTIMORE 1950.

3. WILLIAMS G.H. et BRAUNWALD E. -Hypertension artérielle- Principes de Médecine Interne : 196 : 1024 Médecine-Sciences FLAMMARION PARIS 1989.

4.ACC/AHA/AAPA/ABC/ACPM/AGS/APhA/ASH/ASPC/NMA/PCNA. 2017 Guideline for the Prevention, Detection, Evaluation, and Management of High Blood Pressure in Adults. Report of the American College of Cardiology/American Heart Association Task Force on Clinical Practice Guidelines. Journal of the American college of cardiology vol. 71, no. 19, 2018.

16

Coronary Disease and Heart Infarct

1. MURABITO JM. Women and cardiovascular disease: contributions from the Framingham Heart Study. J Am Med Women's Assoc (1972). 1995 Mar-Apr;50(2):35-9, 55.

2. LESSER M.A. -Testosterone Propionate Therapy in One Hundred Cases of Angina Pectoris: J. Clin. Endocrinol., 6: 549-557, 1946.

3. KRIEG M., SMITH K., and BARTSCH W. -Demonstration of a Specific Androgen Receptor in Rat Heart Muscle: Relationship between Binding Metabolism and Tissue Levels of Androgens: Endocrinology, 103: 1686-1694, 1978.

4. KRIEG M., SMITH K., and ELVERS B. -Androgen Receptor Translocation from Cytosol of Rat Heart Muscle, Bulbocavernosus Levator Ani Muscle and Prostate into heart Muscle Nuclei: J. Steroid Biochem., 13: 577-587, 1980.

5. BLASIUS R., KAFER K., SEITZ W. - Untersuchungen über die Wirkung von Testosteron auf die Contractilen Strukturproteine des Herzens. Klin. Woch., 34, 11/12, 324, 1956.

6. DOMINIQUE SIMON, MARIE-ALINE CHARLES, KHALIL NAHOUL, GENEVIEVE ORSSAUD, JACQUELINE KREJNSKI, VERONIQUE HULLY, EVELYNE JOUBERT, LAURE PAPOZ, AND EVELINE ESCHWEGE. Association between Plasma Total Testosterone and Cardiovascular Risk Factors in Healthy Adult Men: The Telecom Study. Clin. Endocrinol. Metab., 82: 682-685, 1997.

7. KATYA B. RUBINOW, TOMAS VAISAR, CHONGREN TANG, ALVIN M. MATSUMOTO, JAY W. HEINECKE, AND STEPHANIE T. PAGE. Testosterone replacement in hypogonadal men alters the HDL proteome but not HDL cholesterol efflux capacity'" *J. Lipid Res.* 53: 1376-1383, 2012

8. CHEN Y, FU L, HAN Y, TENG Y, SUN J, XIE R, CAO J. Testosterone replacement therapy promotes angiogenesis after acute myocardial infarction by enhancing expression of cytokines HIF-1a, SDF-1a, and VEGF. Eur J Pharmacol. 5; 684(1-3):116-24. 2012 Jun.

9. SIEVERS C, KLOTSCHE J, PIEPER L, SCHNEIDER HJ, MÄRZ W, WITTCHEN HU, STALLA GK, MANTZOROS C. Low testosterone levels predict all-cause mortality and cardiovascular events in women: a prospective cohort study in German primary care patients. Eur J Endocrinol. 2010 Oct;163(4):699-708. Epub 2010 Aug 4.

17

Stiffnesses, Limitation of the Movement, Slipped Discs, and Degenerative Joint Diseases

1. VERZAR F. -Aging of Connective Tissue: Gerontol., 1: 363-378, 1957.

2.VERZAR F. -Studies on Adaptation as a Method of Gerontological Research, in Ciba Colloq. on Aging, 3: 60-72, 1957.

3. ROBERT L. -Les Horloges Biologiques Nouvelle Bibliothèque Scientifique FLAMMARION 1989.

4. SOBEL H. AND MARMORSTON J. Hormonal Influences Upon Connective Tissue Changes of Aging in: PINCUS G (ed.) Recent Progress in Hormone Research, vol. 14. Academic New York 1958.

5. DEBLED G. Hormone stéroïde pour la prévention de maladies associées au vieillissement. OPRI: 100072468. Nº 2019/5905. 13 décembre 2019.

6. SHARON L. HAME, REGINALD A. ALEXANDER. Knee osteoarthritis in women. Curr Rev Musculoskelet Med. 2013 Jun; 6(2): 182–187.

7. MICHELLE J LESPASIO, ASSEM A SULTAN, NICOLAS S PIUZZI, ANTON KHLOPAS, M ELAINE HUSNI, GEORGE F MUSCHLER, MICHAEL A MONT. Hip Osteoarthritis: A Primer. Perm J. 2018; 22: 17-084.

18

Fragile Bones

1. Hormonal Influences Upon Connective Tissue Changes of Aging, SOBEL H. and MARMORSTON J. Institute for Medical Research, Cedars of Lebanon Hospital, and the Department of Biochemistry and Nutrition and the Department of Medicine, University of Southern California, Los Angeles, California, in PINCUS G (ed.) Recent Progress in Hormone Research, vol. 14. Academic New York 1958.

2. RARIY CM, RATCLIFFE SJ, WEINSTEIN R, BHASIN S, BLACKMAN MR, CAULEY JA, ROBBINS J, ZMUDA JM, HARRIS TB, CAPPOLA AR. Higher serum free testosterone concentration in older women is associated with greater bone mineral density, lean body mass, and total fat mass: the cardiovascular health study. J Clin Endocrinol Metab. 2011 Apr;96(4):989-96. Epub 2011 Feb 2.

3. ROSSOUW JE, ANDERSON GL, PRENTICE RL, LACROIX AZ, KOOPERBERG C, et al. Risks and benefits of estrogen plus progestin in healthy postmenopausal women: principal results From the Women's Health Initiative randomized controlled trial. JAMA. 2002; 288:321–333.

4. MORALES-SANTANA S, DÍEZ-PÉREZ A, OLMOS JM, NOGUÉS X, SOSA M, DÍAZ-CURIEL M, PÉREZ-CASTRILLÓN JL, PÉREZ-CANO R, TORRIJOS A, JODAR E, RIO LD, CAEIRO-REY JR, REYES-GARCÍA R, GARCÍA-FONTANA B, GONZÁLEZ-MACÍAS J, MUÑOZ-TORRES M. Circulating sclerostin and estradiol levels are associated with inadequate response to bisphosphonates in postmenopausal women with osteoporosis. Maturitas. Dec;82(4):402-10. 2015

19
Skin Wrinkles

1. MARKUS HAAG, TINA HAMANN, ALEXANDRA E. KULLE, FELIX G. RIEPE, THOMAS BLATT, HORST WENCK, PAUL-MARTIN HOLTERHUS and RETO IVO PEIRANO. Age and skin site-related differences in steroid metabolism in male skin point to a key role of sebocytes in cutaneous hormone metabolism. Dermato-Endocrinology 4 :1, 63-69; January/February/March 2012; ©2012 Landes Bioscience.

22

Kidney Failure

1. DEBLED G. La Pathologie obstructive Congénitale de l'Uretère Terminal. Thèse d'agrégation de l'enseignement supérieur en Sciences Urologiques, Université Libre de Bruxelles, 18 Mai 1971: Acta Urol. Belg., 39: 371-465, 1971

23

Hearing Loss and Vision Troubles

1. CURHAN SG, ELIASSEN AH, EAVEY RD, WANG M, LIN BM, CURHAN GC Menopause and postmenopausal hormone therapy and risk of hearing loss. Menopause. 2017 Sep;24(9):1049-105.

24

Immune Deficiency, Aids, and Cancer

1. SCHUURS A.H.W.M. and VERHEUL H.A.M. -Effects of Gender and Sex Steroids on the Immune Response: J. Steroid Biochem., 35; 2: 157-172, 1990

2. AHMED S.A., PENHALE W.J. and TALAL N. -Sex Hormones, Immune Responses, and Autoimmune Diseases: AJP -121, 3: 531- 551, 1985.

3. SASSON S. and MAYER M. -Antiglucocorticoid Activity of Androgens in Rat Thymus Lymphocytes: Endocrinology, 108: 760-766, 1981.

4. KLEIN SA, KLAUKE S, DOBMEYER JM, DOBMEYER TS, HELM EB, HOELZER H, ROSSOL R. Substitution of testosterone in an HIV-1 positive patient with hypogonadism and Wasting-syndrome led to a reduced rate of apoptosis. Eur J Med Res. 1997 Jan; 2(1):30-2.

5. RODRIGO T. CALADO, WILLIAM T. YEWDELL, KEISHA L. WILKERSON, JOSHUA A. REGAL, SACHIKO KAJIGAYA, CONSTANTINE A. STRATAKIS, AND NEAL S. YOUNG. Sex hormones, acting on the TERT gene, increase telomerase activity in human primary hematopoietic cells. Blood. 2009 Sep 10; 114 (11): 2236-2243.

6. RUSSEL J. REITER, SERGIO A. ROSALES-CORRAL, DUN-XIAN TAN, DARIO ACUNA-CASTROVIEJO, LILAN QIN, SHUN-FA YANG, AND KEXIN XU. Melatonin, a Full-Service Anti-Cancer Agent: Inhibition of Initiation, Progression, and Metastasis. Int J Mol Sci. 2017 Apr; 18(4): 843.

7. DEBLED G. Composition pour le traitement des cancers. OPRI : 100075876. № 2020/5139. 02 mars 2020.

25

Depression

1. OMS. La dépression. Aide-mémoire № 369. October 2012.

2. EHRENKRANZ J., BLISS E., and SHEARD M.H. -Plasma Testosterone: Correlation with Aggressive Behaviour and Social Dominance in Man: Psychosomatic Medicine, 36; 6: 469-475, 1974.

3. KLAIBER E.L., BROVERMAN D.M., VOGEL W., KOBAYASHI Y. -The Use of Steroid Hormones in Depression, in Psychotropic action of hormones: 139 SPECTRUM NEW YORK 1976

4. SELYE HANS. The general adaptation syndrome and the diseases of adaptation. Journal of Allergy. Volume 17, Issue 4, July 1946, Pages 231-247.

5. JENNA MCHENRY, NICOLE CARRIER, ELAINE HULL, AND MOHAMED KABBAJ· Sex differences in anxiety and depression: role of testosterone. Front Neuroendocrinol. 2014 Jan; 35(1): 42–57.

6. KUMSAR Ş, KUMSAR NA, SAĞLAM HS, KÖSE O, BUDAK S, ADSAN Ö. Testosterone levels and sexual function disorders in depressive female

patients: effects of antidepressant treatment. J Sex Med. 2014 Feb;11(2):529-35.

6. KENNETH A. BONNET AND RICHARD P. BROWN in The Biological Role of Dehydroepiandrosterone (DHEA). Walter de Gruyter, Berlin, New York, 1990. p.66-79.

7. JACQUES YOUNG, BEATRICE COUZINET, KHALIL NAHOUL, SYLVIE BRAILLY, PHILIPPE CHANSON, ETIENNE EMILE BAULIEU, AND GILBERT SCHAISON Panhypopituitarism as a Model to Study the Metabolism of Dehydroepiandrosterone (DHEA) in Humans. Journal of Clinical Endocrinology and Metabolism. 82: 2578-2585, 1997

8. R. MORAGA-AMARO, A. VAN WAARDE, J. DOORDUIN, AND E. F. J. DE VRIES. Sex steroid hormones and brain function: PET imaging as a tool for research. J Neuroendocrinol. 2018 Feb; 30(2): e12565.

26

Parkinson's Disease

1. Langston W., PALFREMAN J. The Case of the Frozen Addicts: How the Solution of an Extraordinary Medical Mystery Spawned a Revolution in the Understanding and Treatment of Parkinson's disease. Pantheon Books, New York, 1995.

2. KLAIBER E.L., BROVERMAN D.M., VOGEL W., KOBAYASHI Y. The use of steroid hormones in depression. In Psychotropic action of hormones. Proceedings of the World Congress of biological psychiatry. Buenos Aires. Argentina, September 1974. Spectrum publications INC.

27

Dementias and Alzheimer's Disease

1. Lilly. Press Release Archives. Lilly Announces Top-Line Results of Solanezumab Phase 3 Clinical Trial. Nov 23, 2016.

agrégation2. DEBLED G. Hormone stéroïde pour la prévention de maladies associées au vieillissement. OPRI : 100072468. Nº 2019/5905. 13 décembre 2019.

3. Alzheimer's Association, 2019. Alzheimer's Disease Facts and Figures.

4. RASHAD HUSSAIN, ABDEL M. GHOUMARI, BARTOSZ BIELECKI, JÉRÔME STEIBEL, NELLY BOEHM, PHILIPPE LIERE, WENDY B. MACKLIN, NARENDER KUMAR, RENÉ HABERT, SAKI NA MHAOUTY-KODJA, FRANÇOIS TRONCHE, REGINE SITRUK-WARE, MICHAEL SCHUMACHER, and M. SAID GHANDOUR. The neural androgen receptor: a therapeutic target for myelin repair in chronic demyelination. Brain: 136; 132- 146. May 2013.

5. Dementia. A public Health Priority. WHO report 2012.

6. W. SUE T GRIFFIN, Ph.D., and STEVEN W BARGER, Ph.D. Neuroinflammatory Cytokines-The Common Thread in Alzheimer's Pathogenesis *US Neurol.* 2010: 6(2): 19-27.

7. W. SUE T. GRIFFIN, PH.D. Neuroinflammatory Cytokine Signaling, and Alzheimer's Disease. N Engl J Med 2013; 368:770-771February 21, 2013

8. VOM BERG J, PROKOP S, MILLER KR, OBST J, KÄLIN RE, LOPATEGUI-CABEZAS I, WEGNER A, MAIR F, SCHIPKE CG, PETERS O, WINTER Y, BECHER B, HEPPNER FL. Inhibition of IL-12/IL-23 signaling reduces Alzheimer's disease-like pathology and cognitive decline. Nat Med. 2012 Dec; 18(12): 1812-9.doi: 10.1038/nm.2965. Epub 2012 Nov 25.

9. GUNNAR K. GOURAS, HUAXI XU, RACHEL S. GROSS, JEFFREY P. GREENFIELD, BING HAI, RONG WANG, AND PAUL GREENGARD. Testosterone reduces neuronal secretion of Alzheimer's β-amyloid peptides. Proc Nati Acad Sci U S A. 2000 February 1; 97(3): 1202–1205.

10. GANDY S, ALMEIDA OP, FONTE J, LIM D, WATERRUS A, SPRY N, FLICKER L, MARTINS RN. Chemical andropause and amyloid-beta peptide. JAMA. 2001 May 2; 285(17):2195-6.

11. EMILY R. ROSARIO, Neuroscience Graduate Program, MS. Lilly Chang, MD. Frank Z. Stanczyk, Ph.D. CHRISTIAN J. PIKE, P. Age-Related Testosterone Depletion and the Development of Alzheimer Disease *JAMA. 2004; 292(12):1431-1432.*

12. EMILY R. ROSARIO AND CHRISTIAN J. PIKE. Brain Research Reviews 57, Issue 2, 14 March 2008, Pages 44-453.

13. ROSARIO ER, CHANG L, HEAD EH, STANCZYK FZ, PIKE CJ. Brain levels of sex steroid hormones in men and women during normal aging and in Alzheimer's disease Neurobiol Aging. 2011 Apr ;32(4) :604-13. Epub 2009 May 9.

14. BRADFORD T. WINSLOW, MD, MARY K. ONYSKO, Pharm. D, CHRISTIAN M. STOB, DO, KATHLEEN A. HAZLEWOOD. *Treatment of Alzheimer's Disease. Am Fam Physician.* 2011 Jun 15; 83(12):1403-1412.

15. HIDETAKA OTA, MASAHIRO AKISHITA, TAKUYU AKIYOSHI, TOMOAKI KAHYO, M. ITSUTOSHI SETOU, SUMITO OGAWA, KATSUYA LIJIMA, MASATO ETO, YASUYOSHI OUCHI. Testosterone Deficiency Accelerates Neuronal and Vascular Aging of SAMP8 Mice: Protective Role of eNOS and SIRT1. PLoS ONE I www.plosone.org January 2012 - Volume 7 - Issue 1 - e29598.

16. CHI-FAI LAU, YUEN-SHAN HO, CLARA HIU-LING HUNG, SUTHICHA WUWONGSE, CHUN-HEI POON, KIN CHIU, XIFEI YANG, LEUNG-WING CHU, AND RAYMOND CHUEN-CHUNG CHANG. Protective Effects of Testosterone on Presynaptic Terminals against Oligomeric β-Amyloid Peptide in Primary Culture of Hippocampal Neurons. Hindawi Publishing Corporation. BioMed Research International. Volume 2014, Article ID 103906, 12 pages.

28

Stroke

1. CDC, NCHS. Underlying Cause of Death 1999-2013 on CDCWONDER Online Database2015; e29-322.

Http: Uwonder.cdc.govlycd-jcd10.Html, released in 2015. Data are from the Multiple Cause of Death
Files, 1999-2013, as compiled from data provided by the 57 vital statistics jurisdictions through the
Vital Statistics Cooperative Program. Accessed Feb. 3, 2015.

2. KATHLEEN STRONG CM. RUTH BONITA. Preventing stroke: saving lives around the world. *Lancet Neurol,* vol.6, №2, 2007, p.182-87.

3. MOZAFFARIAN D, BENJAMIN EJ, GO AS, ET AL. Heart disease and stroke statistics-2015 update: a report from the American Heart Association. *Circulation. 2015; e 29-322.*

31

Hormonal Treatment

1. COELINGH BENNINK HJ., HOLINKA CF., and DICZFALUSY E. Estetrol review: profile and potential clinical applications. CLIMACTERIC 2008; II (Suppl I):47-58.

2. COELINGH BENNINK HJT, VERHOEVEN C, ZIMMERMAN Y, VISSER M, FOIDART JM, GEMZELL-DANIELSSON K. Pharmacodynamic effects of the fetal estrogen estetrol in postmenopausal women: results from a multiple-rising-dose study. Menopause: June 2017 - Volume 24 - Issue 6 - p 677–685.

3. SHUSTER, LYNNE T.; RHODES, DEBORAH J.; GOSTOUT, BOBBIE S.; GROSSARDT, BRANDON R.; ROCCA, WALTER A. (2010). "Premature menopause or early menopause: Long-term health consequences." Maturitas. 2010, 65 (2) : 161–166

4. ROSSOUW JE, ANDERSON GL, PRENTICE RL, LACROIX AZ, KOOPERBERG C, et al. Risks and benefits of estrogen plus progestin in healthy postmenopausal women: principal results From the Women's Health Initiative randomized controlled trial. JAMA. 2002; 288:321–333.

5. BERAL V. Breast cancer and hormone-replacement therapy in the Million Women Study. Lancet. 2003; 362:419–427.

6. TJONNELAND A, CHRISTENSEN J, THOMSEN BL, OLSEN A, OVERVAD K, et al. Hormone replacement therapy in relation to breast carcinoma incidence: a prospective Danish cohort study. Cancer. 2004; 100:2328–2337.

7. MAGNUSSON C, BARON JA, CORREIA N, BERGSTROM R, ADAMI HO, et al. Breast-cancer risk following long-term estrogen- and estrogen-progestin-replacement therapy. Int J Cancer. 1999; 81:339–344.

8. STAHLBERG C, PEDERSEN AT, LYNGE E, ANDERSEN ZJ, KEIDING N, et al. Increased risk of breast cancer following different regimens of hormone replacement therapy frequently used in Europe. Int J Cancer. 2004; 109:721–727.

9. FUGH-BERMAN A, MCDONALD CP, BELL AM, BETHARDS EC, SCIALLI AR. Department of Physiology and Biophysics, Georgetown University Medical Center, Washington, DC, USA. The promotional tone in reviews of menopausal hormone therapy after the Women's Health Initiative: an analysis of published articles. PLoS Med. 2011 Mar;8(3): e1000425. Epub 2011 Mar 15.

10. KANG WANG, FENG LI, LI CHEN, YAN-MEI LAI, XIANG ZHANG, and HONG-YUAN LI. Change in the risk of breast cancer after receiving hormone replacement therapy by considering effect-modifiers: a systematic review and dose-response meta-analysis of prospective studies. Oncotarget. 2017 Oct 6; 8(46): 81109–81124.

11. XUEZHI (DANIEL) JIANG, MD, Ph.D. *et al.* Significantly higher' side effects with pellet vs. FDA-approved HT. P-50. Presented at: Annual Meeting of the North American Menopause Society; Oct. 11-14, 2017; Philadelphia

12. BASSON Rosemary. Testosterone therapy to reduced libido in women. Therapeutic advances in endocrinology and metabolism 1(4):155-64 · August 2010 - Article (PDF Available).

13. ANDREY V DOLINKO and ELIZABETH S GINSBURG. Hyperandrogenism in menopause: a case report and literature review. Fertil Res Pract. 2015; 1: 7.

14. DEBLED G. The menopausal disease. Approaches to aging control: 19:17-24, October 2015.

15. DEBLED G. L'Andropause, cause, conséquences et remèdes. Maloine, Paris, 1988.

16. DEBLED G: Ageless Man. HMS WORLD Editions, 2017

17. DEBLED G. The androgenic disease of andropause. SEMAL congress, Seville, October 5, 2019.

18. DEBLED G. Mesterolone pharmaceutical composition for dihydrotestosterone deficiencies in the woman. EPO. Application N° Patent N° 121/6851.9 - 1466/268/215 European Patent Bulletin 18/48 of 28.11.18.

19. DEBLED G. Hormone stéroïde pour la prévention de maladies associées au vieillissement. OPRI: 100072468. Nº 2019/5905. 13 décembre 2019.

CPSIA information can be obtained
at www.ICGtesting.com
Printed in the USA
LVHW081437160621
690385LV00007B/494